DYNAMICS OF LAW
IN NURSING
AND HEALTH CARE

DYNAMICS OF LAW
IN NURSING
AND HEALTH CARE

Mary Delores Hemelt, R.N., B.S.N., M.S., J.D.

Chairman, Board of Review,
Maryland State Department of Mental Health & Hygiene
Practicing Attorney
Professor, Essex Community College

Mary Ellen Mackert, B.S., R.N., B.S.N., M.S.N.

President, Health Care Workshops
Nursing Consultant
Professor, Harford Community College

Reston Publishing Company
A Prentice-Hall Company
Reston, Virginia

Library of Congress Cataloging in Publication Data

Hemelt, Mary Dolores
   Dynamics of law in nursing and health care.

   Bibliography:
   Includes index.
    1. Medical laws and legislation—United States.
2. Nursing—Law and legislation—United States.
I. Mackert, Mary Ellen, joint author. II. Title.
[DNLM: 1. Jurisprudence—United States—Nursing texts.
2. Delivery of health care—United States—Nursing
texts. WY33 AA1 H4d]
KF3821.H46   344′.73′041   77-28976
ISBN 0-87909-208-4

© 1978 by Reston Publishing Company, Inc.
A Prentice-Hall Company
Reston, Virginia 22090

10 9 8 7 6 5

Printed in the United States of America

This book is lovingly dedicated to Joe and Margaret

Contents

Part One   Dynamic Law Applied to Health Care   2

Dynamics of Law   3
   Introduction   3
   Adversary Proceeding   4
   Origin of Law   5
   Intentional Torts   7
   Tort   10
   Standard of Reasonableness   10
   Negligence   11
   Cause of Action   13
   Weight of Evidence   17

Doctrines and Principles of Law   18
   Legal Expectations   18
   Specific Doctrines and Principles of Law   22
   Doctrine of Personal Liability   22
   Doctrine of Respondeat Superior   24
   Doctrine of Borrowed Servant   26
   Doctrine of the Reasonably Prudent Man   28
   Doctrine of Corporate Negligence   31

Doctrine of Res Ipsa Loquitur   34
Doctrine of Foreseeability   36
Doctrine of Outrageous Conduct or *Tort of Emotional
    Distress*   39

Defenses and Damages   40
Contributory Negligence   41
Comparative Negligence   41
Statute of Limitations   42
Types of Damages   43

Contracts   44
Definition of a Contract   44
Elements of a Contract   45
Breach of Contract and Remedies   46
Classifications of Contracts   48
Contracts and Patients   48
Contracts with Employers   49
Case on Contracts   52
Labor Relations—Why Do Persons Organize,
    or Join a Union?   53
Collective Bargaining Under the National Labor Relations Act
    and Amendments   53

Part Two   Contemporary Legal-Medical Issues   60

Evolution of the Right to Health Care   61
Courts and Health Care Rights   62
Health Care Delivery System and Patient's Rights   62
Contemporary Issues   63
Self Evident Rights and Rights in General   64

Abortion   68
Arguments Related to Abortion   68
Decisions on Abortion   69

Child Abuse   72
Definition of Child Abuse   72
History   72
Beginning Legislation   73
Distinction Between Abuse and Neglect   74
Profile of a Child Abuser   75
Public Education   78

Some Indications of Child Abuse   78
Conclusion   79
Case of Child Abuse   79

Dignified Death   81
Sanctity of Life   83
What is Death?   84
Death by Choice   85
Making the Decision   88

The Patient's Right to Know   90
Doctrine of Informed Consent   90
Who May Consent   92
Informed Consent   94
Liability of the Nurse   97
Consent to Transsexual or Sex-Reassignment Surgery   98
Case on Doctrine of Informed Consent   99

Involuntary Commitment   101
Emergency Admission and Non-Emergency Admission   101
Admission of Minors to Mental Health Care Agencies   103

Confidentiality   104
Definition of Privacy   104
Right of Privacy   105
Permissible Disclosure of Medical Information   107
Liability for Disclosure of Confidential Information   108
Distinction Between Confidential Communication and
    Privileged Communication   111

Medical Records   112
Nurses Notes   114
Alteration   118
Access to Medical Records   119
Summary   120

Part Three   Vignettes   122

Introduction to Vignettes   123
Vignettes:
1. Confidentiality and Computer Information Data   124
2. Medication Refusal   126
3. Restraints   128

4. Staff Relationships, Affiliating Students   131
5. Countersigning   133
6. Informed Consent   135
7. Informed Consent Situation   136
8. Illegible Orders   138
9. Leaving Against Medical Advice   139
10. Employee Relationships   141
11 Inadequate Care and Incompetent Staff   143
12. Privacy Case   145
13. Resuscitation   146
14. Denying Heroic Measures   148
15. Teaching Hospitals   150
16. Splitting Medication   152
17. Contract   153
18. Defective Equipment   155
19. Supervision   156
20. Staffing   158
21. Communications   160
22. Pharmacy   162
23. Protecting Personal Property   164
24. Wills   166
24A. Wills—Signature   170
25. Insurance Situation   171
26. Teaching Cardiopulmonary Resuscitation to L.P.N.'s
and Aides   174
27. Labor Relations Situation   175
28. Workmen's Compensation Case   178
29. Police Powers Situation   178
30. Contributory Negligence or Comparative
Negligence Situation   180
31. Medication Administration   182
32. Search and Seizure   183

Guidelines and Closing Comments   187
Conclusion   189

Part Four   Appendices   190

Appendix I   History   191
Appendix II   Classifications of Law Affecting Health
Care Professionals   192
Appendix III   Court System   195
Appendix IV   Authority   200

Part Five   Evaluation of Processed Content   204

    Section A Definitions   205
    Section B True/False Items   205
    Section C Multiple Choice Items   207
    Section D Situations   211
      Answers   217

Glossary   220

Bibliography   236

Index   244

Foreword

There are several excellent textbooks on the legal responsibilities of health care practitioners. However, this text represents a significant departure from others by 1) presenting the basic theories and principles of law utilized in the medical-legal field, and 2) applying those principles to the "real world" situations.

The premise on which this book is based is that practitioners of health care are faced with critical daily decisions in providing quality health care to their patients. These decisions place the decision-makers in a position of legal accountability and possible liability.

This material has obviously been written to aid nurses and other health care practitioners to make appropriate decisions in their daily practice. The text as written is a pragmatic approach to develop a systematic effort in acquiring, developing and maintaining the knowledge, and beginning analytical skills to meet legal responsibilities and avoid legal liabilities.

This book is grounded in practicality. It is my conviction that theory not significantly related to application is non-meaningful. It is the theory and basic principles of law that give us the foundation for legal and appropriate action.

I believe the design, style, and content of this text will have a profound influence on health care. The authors have made a substantial contribution to the health care of patients and the professional lives of those who care for patients.

Mary M. Jerome, R.N., B.S.
Associate Chief

Preface

The health profession is extremely concerned with lawsuits and litigation in everyday practice in the health setting. In some instances, health care practitioners are semi-paralyzed in functioning because of concern over being sued by their patients. Much of the fear is from misunderstanding and misinformation. In this text, the term *health care practitioner* is used in a broad sense to connote persons dealing directly with patients. Although much of the book concerns nurses, the principles and information contained herein are applicable to physicians, physicians assistants, laboratory technicians and other allied health personnel. Therefore, whenever the term health care practitioner is used, it is to be interpreted in the broadest definition.

Dynamics of Law in Nursing and Health Care is intended for use as a resource to all workers in the health field. It is meant to be a guide to assist them in their responsibilities to the patient, to the employer, and to themselves. It is hoped that it will compensate those readers who have received inadequate information regarding their possible liabilities and responsibilities in their working hours.

This book is more than a revision of others in the field. The intent is to give, in simplified language, an overview of the medical-legal problems, and explain how the health practitioner can protect himself from being sued, or worse yet, from being found liable.

The authors have attempted to demonstrate the dynamics of law in the daily events of health issues and to show how extensive the relationship is between the fields of law and medicine.

The authors are cognizant of the changing scene in health delivery and present some of the recent developments. The emphasis of this text is to determine the authority for an individual's action in a given set of circumstances and to determine one's own liability for one's acts in a particular set of circumstances.

Part One deals with the dynamics of law and the doctrines and principles of law. It lays the foundation for an understanding of various legal issues in today's health care world. Included is a section on contracts because contractual agreements are so much a part of one's professional life. Following are sections on organizing and labor relations. The authors do not present a pro or con union statement, but rather a statement of the importance of cohesiveness and unity in the health care profession.

Part Two deals with contemporary ethical-legal issues involving patient's rights. Specific attention is focused on the issues of abortion, child abuse, dignified death, right to be informed, involuntary commitment, confidentiality and medical records.

Part Three is designed to assist the reader in implementing learning of the textbook material. This unique adjunct presents a variety of common work situations in which the reader might be involved in professional life. These situations are termed *vignettes*. Each vignette is followed by a suggested answer. The intention of the authors is to give the reader an opportunity to formulate a rational, legal solution to the work situation by identifying the main issue to be answered and selecting the doctrines or principles of law that apply. This method assists the reader to implement and process the informational material learned in earlier chapters. The purpose of the vignettes is to convince the reader that action based on ethical, managerial and legal principles will lead to appropriate action and decrease the risk of legal liability.

Part Four, the appendices, contains information on the history and classifications of law, the court system, and the concept of authority. These sections give background information on topics referred to earlier in the text.

Part Five comprises text items designed to determine if certain information was processed by the reader. Included are true-false items, multiple choice items and definition of terms used in the text. Brief situations are presented for the reader to consider the legal implications involved. The test answers follow at the end of the section.

It should be recognized by all who use the book that the law is an adversary system. There are no absolute right and wrong answers to be given to the situation presented. When this is understood, the reader will be able to apply the principles set forth and process them accordingly, making applications of these principles to his own environment or work situation.

Throughout the book, you will note that the bottom of many pages contains words which are defined. These are words not commonly understood by those outside the legal profession. This will help you to more clearly understand the material presented. A glossary of terms is also available at the end of the book.

The authors have presented educational programs concerning legal aspects of health care on a local, state, and national level. A collection of hundreds of the work situation problems was made as demonstrated by the participants. The vignettes in this textbook represent problems most frequently presented by participants from major cities across the United States. During the collection process, research showed repeated concern over the issues of informed consent, restraints, resuscitation, verbal orders, scope of practice, confidentiality, staffing shortage, responsibility for peers or co-workers, and assuming pharmacy responsibilities. These issues formed the core for development of the vignettes—specific situations with specific answers. It should be understood that no attempt was made to develop a vignette for every subject discussed in the text. Rather, they were developed to cover different subjects in various categories.

An important contribution from the authors is to demonstrate how important the law is in ways not yet appreciated by the reader, and to motivate the reader to watch for daily issues in the health field and look for future implications. Naturally, the authors concede that no textbook, however well intentioned, can substitute for legal consultation in appropriate circumstances.

The authors wish to thank Diane Breunig Freed for her editorial supervision during the production of this book.

Mary Dolores Hemelt

Mary Ellen Mackert

DYNAMICS OF LAW
IN NURSING
AND HEALTH CARE

Part One
DYNAMIC LAW APPLIED TO HEALTH CARE

DYNAMICS OF LAW

Introduction

Law is the sum total of rules and regulations by which society is governed. It is man-made and it regulates social conduct in a formal and binding manner. It reflects society's needs, attitudes, and mores. A simple society requires few rules, but a complex society requires a complicated legal framework for guidance and survival. This set of established rules makes it easier for people to live with one another, and it affects us every day whether or not we realize it.

The law, however, is not rigidly fixed, but a composite of court decisions, state and federal statutes, regulations and procedures. Interpretations of diverse state laws by different courts or small variations in the circumstances of a case may lead to very different conclusions in two seemingly similar situations. You will soon discover there are no final answers. Law is dynamic—it lives, grows, and changes. No book or set of books, no lawyer or teacher can tell you with complete assurance what is right or wrong or what the final outcome of any case will be.

For example, in the *Doe v. Poelker* (515 F.2d 541 (1973)) case, the courts held that an indigent patient seeking an abortion in a municipal hospital was entitled to that abortion under the law. The court prohibited the mayor from making policy that would interfere with an indigent patient's right to an abortion. In June of 1977 the Supreme Court of the United States ruled that nothing in the Social Security Act or the U.S. Constitution entitled the indigent patient to free abortions. Congress is presently working on new legislation to clarify and identify which patients, if any, should receive consideration in light of the Supreme Court ruling.

The realistic approach to this paradox is that, at best, you have only general principles of law to apply to a set of facts. This situation, understandably, often distresses individuals because they are much more comfortable with specific answers to questions and issues.

The legislatures in every state throughout the United States and the Congress pass new laws daily. The courts in every state and the Supreme Court of the United States make decisions through the judicial process that change some aspect of our legal system. It is comparable to the continuous revision of health care procedures, or the proliferation of new drugs on the market. Certainly one recognizes that the health care field is constantly changing as new techniques and procedures are adopted almost daily. However, certain principles of health care never change. The principle of sterile technique and the need for it to be applied in caring for patients to prevent infection is generally applicable for all patients. Analogous to this are the general principles of law which can be applied to one's daily work situations. This application of the principles of law and the case law, as it is known at the time, to a work situation will usually result in an appropriate legal response. It is necessary to act within the framework of the law at the particular time one is reviewing the facts; that is how one is expected to conduct oneself.

Adversary Proceeding

The American courts, which have their basis in the English court system, follow what is called an *adversary proceeding*. This is a confrontation between two parties with each side selecting the "strongest" supporters for his cause. There are certain rules to be followed and certain conduct is prescribed. The forum is on neutral ground and the rules and procedures have been prepared with the hope that truth will be defined and justice realized once the parties verbally and figuratively clash—each hoping to prevail in the end.

The system has been criticized with some justification at times; however, no one has yet found a better method of obtaining truth than by subjecting an individual to cross-examination by a skilled attorney. When the appropriate questions are asked, rephrased and asked again,

Justice: the constant and perpetual disposition to render every man his due

or when a defect in the consistency of testimony has been detected and exploited, *justice* is usually served.

The famous Watergate hearings permitted the American public to observe a Senatorial Committee questioning witnesses. It was not unusual to observe a witness testifying and appearing to be the epitome of truthfulness and integrity. However, often upon reexamination by another senator or when comparing previous testimony before another tribunal, inconsistencies in statements and even outright contradictions could be detected.

Although the Watergate hearings were not judicial proceedings (which normally would be guided by stricter rules of evidence and procedures), they served to demonstrate to the public the benefit of questions and point out why the courts have followed the adversary proceeding method to get at the truth of certain matters.

Francis L. Wellman in *The Art of Cross-examination* explains that what each person sees, hears, and believes to be fact will differ from the neutral, objective happening based on each individual's frame of reference. Knowledge is only the impression of one's mind and not the fact itself. The stimulus is always the same. Variance arises when the sensation is interpreted by the individual and becomes a perception. This interpretation of a sensation is a personal and individual act and varies according to previous experiences and various characteristics. Therefore different individuals can perceive the same stimulus differently.

The court system has been derived precisely because reasonable men can differ as to the inferences and conclusions to be drawn from facts as perceived by them. Here the judge, or judge and jury, listen to the presentation of both sides, observe their demeanor, examine any documents or exhibits presented, and attempt to render an objective opinion based on evidence which is as factual as possible.

Origin of Law

Law refers to those man-made rules which regulate social conduct in a formal and legally binding manner. Both statutory and common law are of equal importance and legal effect.

Laws regulating human social conduct are derived from two basic sources. One source finds expression in formal legislative enactments generally referred to as *statutes* or statutory law; for example, law passed by Congress or a state legislative body. Thus, the distinguishing feature of statutory law is that it is derived from formal legislative enactments. Since legislative bodies cannot possibly enact statutes to cover all types of human conduct, there are gaps in the law which must be filled by the second basic source of law, that is, judicial decisions which interpret legal issues raised in disputes taken to court. This judge-made law, referred to as *common law*, is distinguished from the more formal type of law expressed in legislative enactments.

Restated, statutory law is enacted by a legislative body, while common law is derived from court decisions.

Criminal and Civil Law   Although law can be classified in many different ways, it is sufficient for us to deal with the two major classifications—criminal law and civil law. Criminal law deals with conduct considered offensive to society as a whole. An act which is expressly prohibited by statutory or common law is called a *crime*. The punishment for committing a crime is imprisonment or a fine.

The general concept of a crime is that it is an act done in an evil way. This is not entirely true. Certain acts are crimes because they are prohibited by public policy. Although the act which constitutes the crime may be done on or against an individual citizen, it is viewed as an act or crime against society as a whole and not against the individual citizen. Therefore, it is society who prosecutes the defendant and the legal proceeding is in the name of the people, e.g., State versus John Doe.

There are specific elements that constitute a crime. Every element must be established before an individual can be charged and convicted of a crime. Those elements must be proven in a court of law by evidence and proof. This evidence and proof must be established beyond a reasonable doubt and with a moral certainty before the defendant charged with the crime can be found guilty. It would be impossible and impractical to do more than generalize regarding the elements which constitute crimes. The elements for any crime, such as failure to report a gunshot wound or a contagious disease to the proper authorities, are spelled out in the statute precisely and exactly. Two conditions common to all crimes, however, are criminal intent and an overt positive or negative act in violation of the specific law. When an individual is charged with a crime, it is necessary to establish that the individual intended to commit the crime with which he is charged. The intention can be inferred by the act or imputed to the individual because the action or inaction is declared a crime. In those cases it is not necessary to establish a criminal intent by additional evidence.

Crime: a positive or negative act in violation of a law forbidding or requiring it; an offense against the state

Examples where violation of a required act constitutes a crime and intent is inferred by law are the practice of medicine and nursing without a license. In other types of crimes, such as murder or manslaughter, evidence to establish the existence of a criminal intent is necessary. But because intent is a subjective mental state, the judge and jury may conclude from the act performed by the defendant and the circumstances surrounding the action or inaction that there was criminal intent. Therefore, even if the actor performing a crime was motivated by good intentions, it is still both reasonable and possible to conclude that the defendant charged had criminal intent when looking at the totality of circumstances. For example, if a nurse intending to alleviate a patient's pain gave a wrong dose of medication which resulted in the patient's death, she could be charged with involuntary manslaughter.

The second major class of law, *civil law*, is concerned with the legal rights and duties of private persons, in contrast to criminal law which is concerned with public rights and public authority to punish for unlawful conduct.

To explain more clearly, let us use the example of assault and battery. This is a cause of action, which really is both a criminal act and a civil act. So, in effect, if someone were beaten by John Doe, and assuming the facts to be true, John Doe would be guilty of a criminal act of assault and battery as well as a civil act of assault and battery. Therefore, he could be fined and imprisoned for the crime and the victim would have a right to a civil action for redress in money damages from John Doe. In fact, even though the victim may later wish to drop all charges, the crime of criminal assault remains. It is a public crime against society. As such, the state has been injured and must therefore protect the public by punishing the individual.

Intentional Torts

There are certain specific torts known as *intentional torts* that are distinguished from the tort of negligence. Some of these specific torts

Murder: unlawful killing of a human being by another with malice aforethought, either expressed or implied

Manslaughter: unlawful killing of another without malice, either expressed or implied, either voluntarily or involuntarily, in the commission of an unlawful act

Cause of action: averment of allegations or facts sufficient to cause the defendant to respond to allegations

are assault and battery, false imprisonment, defamation, invasion of privacy, and fraud. They are distinguished from the tort of negligence because the plaintiff must establish that the defendant intended to commit the specific wrong alleged. These torts are more serious than acts of negligence. As a result, punitive as well as actual damages may be awarded.

The intention to commit the tort can be established by the proof of an objective act from which certain inferences that the actor knew or should have known that a certain result would follow the act can be drawn. For conduct to be construed as intentional, there must be the conscious performance of an act to accomplish a specific result, or where a reasonable person would know that a particular consequence of the act would occur. Therefore, to be intentional the act must be both deliberate and conscious. As indicated, the distinguishing element in intentional torts is *intent*. As legally defined it need not be hostile. In fact, most health care practitioners could be acting with good intentions, but if they invade a legally protected interest of the patient it may lead to charges of intentional tort.

Assault and Battery   The law protects individuals from unpermitted and unprivileged contact to his person. If a patient has refused a particular hypodermic injection and the nurse approaches the patient and attempts to administer the medication, it would be an *assault*. If the nurse administers the hypodermic injection, it would be a *battery*. The essence of the assault is the threat and the apparent ability to carry out the threat to touch the patient without his consent. The battery is the assault carried out or completed. Therefore, the patient must be conscious for an assault to occur. An unconscious patient may be the victim of a battery. Thus, performing surgery or a procedure on an unconscious patient without his consent is a battery. It is not an assault because the patient is not aware of the threat to his person. The basis for the liability for the battery is the lack of consent to the body contact.

There are certain circumstances where an individual committing a battery will not be liable for the battery. These are situations in which the conduct is said to be privileged. For example, a nurse restraining a patient who is obviously about to strike or injure other patients would be acting appropriately. The action of the nurse to protect other patients and their interests outweighs the damage that

Assault: threatening to do bodily harm
Battery: committing bodily harm

may be sustained by the restraining of the patient and his interest. The restriction on the striking patient should be limited to that which is necessary to protect the other patients and should not be extended wihout sufficient basis or need to do so.

False Imprisonment The tort of *false imprisonment* refers to the conscious restraint of the freedom of another individual without proper authorization, privilege or consent of the individual restrained. The confinement must be intentional and without legal justification. Freedom from unlawful restraint is a right protected by law. If a patient is improperly restrained, the law allows redress in the form of damages for this tort. The proof of all the elements of false imprisonment must be established to sustain that an illegal act was done. In situations where patients are a danger to themselves or to others, the patient may be restrained. However, the restraint must be limited to and in proportion to the exigencies of need to be restrained and is based on reasonableness. What would a reasonable prudent health practitioner do in such circumstances? This is the standard. If the patient's conduct is such that reasonable persons would believe the patient will injure himself or others, the restraint would be proper and privileged.

Defamation of Character *Defamation of character* is a communication about another person which exposes that person to contempt or diminishes his reputation. The written defamation is termed *libel*. The oral defamation is termed *slander*. These are torts that affect the reputation and good name of another. The statements must be communicated to a second party. The basic element of the tort of defamation is that the oral or written communication is made to another person other than the one defamed. In general, truth is a defense to charges of defamation. Also there are certain situations that are considered privileged. For example, head nurses or supervisors who must evaluate employees or give references regarding an employee's work have a qualified privilege. This means the law recognizes that certain relationships require an individual be allowed to speak without fear of being sued for defamation of character. They are not subject to actions of defamation for making bona fide evaluations of their employees. Evaluations made in good faith and without any malice, even if later proved wrong, are not actionable, if reasonable under the circumstances.

Exigency: state of requiring immediate aid or attention
Redress: receiving satisfaction from an injury sustained

Invasion of Privacy and Confidentiality are discussed in Part 2 of the text.

Fraud *Fraud* is defined as the intentional perversion of truth for the purpose of inducing another to rely on it and part with something of value or surrender a legal right. The elements that constitute the intentional tort of fraud are 1) the fraud is willful and intentional, 2) the fraud must attach to material misrepresentation, 3) the misstatement must be known to be untrue, and 4) the fraud causes a loss or harm to the victim. The plaintiff who alleges that a fraud has been perpetrated on him has the burden of proving all the elements of fraud. Misrepresentations of matters of fact can occur where a patient has received a wrong medication or treatment and this matter is concealed from the patient. This type of action on the part of the nurse or anyone else that misleads or deliberately deceives the patient is improper. It is negligent conduct to give a patient a wrong medication or treatment, but it is fraudulent conduct to cover up errors and more serious in the eyes of the law. The patient is entitled to the truth. Negligence, of course, is not condoned. But mistakes do happen. It is understandable that errors can occur in the complex health care system. It is not understandable that patients would be deceived about such errors. Judges and juries can appreciate the pressures that health care practitioners are under that sometimes result in injury to patients. Judges and juries cannot appreciate fraudulent conduct and they deal with this type of conduct more harshly.

Tort

The general category of civil law with which health professionals are concerned is called the law of torts. A *tort* is a legal or civil wrong committed by one person against the person or property of another. To compensate for such a private legal wrong, the court will provide a remedy in the form of an action for damages. The law permits the harmed person to bring a civil action against the wrongdoer to recover a sum of money as redress or compensation for the injury suffered. Therefore, a tort is a civil wrong for which the court will provide a remedy in the form of an action for damages.

Standard of Reasonableness

The common thread woven into all torts is the idea of unreasonable interference with the interest of others. It seems that liability is based on conduct which is socially unreasonable. This is the dilemma you will be facing. What is unreasonable social conduct? There is no exact answer. The balance known as "reasonable" is undoubtedly somewhere between the plaintiff's claim to protection against damage and the defendant's claims to freedom of action. It is the inherent right of every individual to expect individuals to use reasonable care in their dealings with one another. The definition of *reasonable care* in regard to health care practitioners is generally understood as this:

> That degree of skill and knowledge customarily used by a competent health practitioner of similar education and experience in treating and caring for the sick and injured in the community in which the individual is practicing or learning his profession.

For example, it is reasonable to expect that a nurse working with a patient who is in a leg cast would check the leg to see that there is proper circulation. Whether the doctor orders certain observations or not, it is incumbent on every nurse to make the necessary observations to assure the limb is not subjected to impaired circulation. It is common knowledge to health care practitioners that any extremity with impaired circulation for any length of time can result in irreversible ischemia. Therefore, a nurse who failed to make these types of observations would not be giving "reasonable care" and would fall below the standard required.

Negligence

Negligence law is a broad field which includes many types of negligent conduct in carrying out one's legal responsibilities to others. In law, every person is always responsible for conducting himself in a reasonable and prudent manner, whether he is a layman or a professional and whether he is engaged in the simplest or most complex type of activity. When a person fails to conduct himself in the prescribed manner and thereby does harm to another, the law says he is legally *negligent*. It embraces the area commonly referred to as *malpractice law* and includes the negligent conduct of physicians, dentists, nurses, pharmacists, engineers, lawyers, architects, and other professionally trained persons. Thus, malpractice is concerned with the negligent conduct of all professional persons.

Now that you are aware of the general relationship between tort law, negligence law, and malpractice law, let us analyze the concept of negligence in more detail. The term "negligence" as used in malpractice law is not necessarily the same as "carelessness." While conduct which is careless is usually negligent, conduct can also be held negligent in the legal sense even if one acts carefully. Acting carefully and acting negligently are not necessarily mutually exclusive. For example, if a health practitioner attempts a procedure for which he or she has had no prior training and does it carefully, the conduct, nevertheless, can be deemed negligent if harm results to the patient because the practitioner attempted the procedure without having had previous training or experience. The fact that the practitioner was careful in carrying out the procedure is considered immaterial from the legal standpoint.

Liability   Liability is not an easy concept to grasp. A health practitioner's careful conduct may still be legally negligent if what is performed (even though it is done with great care) is not what other prudent health practitioners would have done in the same circumstances. This assumes that some harm results from the health practitioner's act, for without harm resulting, no legal wrong (tort) has been committed. Generally, careful conduct will not give rise to a charge of negligence, but it brings up the term *liability*. When we say that an individual is legally liable to another person because of the individual's negligent conduct, we mean he can be held legally responsible for the harm caused the other person. *Liability* refers to the state of being held legally liable. In a malpractice action (as in other civil actions), liability is assessed in monetary terms, commonly referred to as either *money damages* or simply *damages*.

Another point to remember is that a negligent act committed by a professional person constitutes malpractice only if it involves negligence in the carrying out of his professional duties. Medical malpractice is that type of malpractice which relates specifically to the acts of health care professionals when they are carrying out their normal patient care responsibilities. In other words, medical malpractice is negligence in some aspect of medical care and treatment.

Classification of Malpractice   There are three classifications of malpractice.

1. Criminal malpractice includes such crimes as assault and battery or euthansia.

Standard of care: skill and learning commonly possessed by members of the profession

2. Civil malpractice includes that practice which falls below a reasonable standard and which amounts to a breach of professional competence to the patient.
3. Ethical malpractice includes violations of professional ethics which result in censure or disciplinary actions by professional associations or licensing boards.

Cause of Action

As stated previously, a tort is a civil wrong against an individual.

In order to have a cause of action based on negligence or malpractice, the following four elements must be shown to exist:

1. There was a duty owed to the plaintiff by the defendant to use due care.
2. The duty was breached by the defendant by being negligent.
3. The plaintiff was injured or damaged in some way.
4. The plaintiff's injury was caused by the defendant's negligence.

That is, the proximate cause of the patient's injury must be the defendant's negligence. There must be a causal connection between the plaintiff's injury and the defendant's action. (See Exhibit 1.) All four elements of a tort must be clearly developed or there can be no recovery in tort.

The plaintiff must establish that a health practitioner/patient relationship existed. The plaintiff must establish what the standard of care is for health practitioners in the same locale and with similar education and skills. This is critical to the case. Failure to establish the standard of care could result in the plaintiff's not being permitted to go forward with the case. After establishing the standard of care, the plaintiffs must show that the defendant failed to meet it. The plaintiff must establish that the injury to him was a direct result of the defendant's failure to maintain the standard of care. The plaintiff must make a monetary claim for compensation for injury and damages.

Due care: reasonable care under the circumstances
Proximate cause: legal concept of cause and effect, the injury would not have occurred but for the particular cause

---

CAUSE OF ACTION OR PRIMA FACIE CASE

4 D's

1. Duty Owed
2. Duty Breached
3. Damages
4. Direct cause or Proximate cause

Exhibit 1.

These damages include pain and suffering, loss of wages, medical fees and other costs related to the injury.

Whether the relationship between the plaintiff and defendant was such that there was a clear obligation of due care owed by the defendant is a question of law for the court to decide. The questions of whether the defendant was negligent, whether the plaintiff was actually injured, and whether the defendant's negligence caused the injury to the plaintiff are all questions of fact for a jury to decide. From the evidence presented, the jury comes to a conclusion about what in fact happened. The judge then applies the law of the state to the conclusion of the jury. In a negligence case, the fact that the defendant's injury to the plaintiff is unintentional is immaterial and does not change the tort of negligence. It is important to realize that when the plaintiff has suffered no injury, he has no cause of action; therefore, the defendant cannot be guilty of negligence. For example, a doctor may order penicillin for a patient with a known allergy to the drug and the health practitioner may administer the medication without checking the patient's known allergies. But if the patient has no reaction to the drug at this particular time, there is no injury, hence no cause of action.

It is essential at law that all four elements for a cause of action be present to establish sufficient facts to cause the *allegations* charged to be answered. If any one of the elements is not established, there is no cause of action. This is basic to the initiation of a suit. It does not establish negligence or non-negligence. It does not mean the plaintiff will win his case. It simply means that the plaintiff has established certain factors from which reasonable men could presume he was injured and the defendant negligently caused those injuries. As a result of establishing these factors, the plaintiff has a legal right to sue the defendant and force the defendant to answer the allegations made by the plaintiff. The defendant must be given the opportunity to rebut the charges with witnesses and evidence. This, in essence, establishes a prima facie case for malpractice. It should be noted that the law expects a plaintiff to minimize his loss by exercise of ordinary care.

Therefore, a patient who has suffered a loss cannot recover for additional loss or injury which he could have prevented by ordinary prudence. This, of course, would be a reasonable expectation. At the same time, when any individual causes a tortuous injury to another individual, that individual is responsible for all the results of that particular injury.

Civil Suit Procedure   Basically, the lawyer attempts to establish a legal basis for the plaintiff's claim against health professionals. The investigator (lawyer) looks at each set of circumstances surrounding a claim reviewed and asks the question, "Is there legally sufficient evidence to make a prima facie case that the plaintiff has a justifiable reason to place a suit against a defendant?" *Prima facie evidence,* according to Black's Dictionary of Law, is such evidence that is sufficient to establish a given fact, or a group or chain of facts, constituting a party's claim of defense, if not rebutted or contradicted is sufficient for the plaintiff's case. The plaintiff is felt to have a *prima facie case* when the evidence in his favor is sufficiently strong for the defendant to be called upon to answer the plaintiff's allegation. The only time a defendant is legally negligent is when a judge or jury finds him so in a stated verdict.

Lawsuits are structured affairs, conducted in accordance with written rules. The need for rules is self-evident. Courts are concerned with two main functions: 1) to resolve disputes between parties in a way consistent with the applicable law and principles of justice, and 2) to accomplish this within a time frame that will make the relief granted meaningful. In its broad aspects, the course of a civil action can be traced through several distinct procedures or steps. These are the following:

1. filing of complaint by plaintiff against defendant
2. response of defendant, termed answer
3. pretrial activities of both parties to elicit all the facts in a situation, termed *discovery*
4. the trial of the case in which all relevant facts are presented to judge and/or jury
5. jury decision
6. appeal from decision by losing party.

The complaint is drafted after the plaintiff's attorney evaluates the cause of action, the legal rules that have been violated, and the

Prima facie case: on its face, first appearance

amount of damages suffered by the plaintiff. The complaint is filed in court and a copy served on the defendant. The complaint has certain purposes. It notifies the defendant that he is being sued, and it tells the defendant in greater detail why he is being sued. It spells out the allegations.

The defendant should seek legal counsel and answer the complaint no matter how unfair it may seem; otherwise the court presumes the plaintiff's complaint is true and orders relief. The defendant may admit some allegations and deny others in the complaint. Generally, the defendant disagrees with the plaintiff's characterization of the incident and sets forth defenses in his answer of response. For example, the defendant may deny all charges, the defendant may allege the plaintiff contributed to the accident, or the defendant may argue that the statute of limitations has expired. This means that the time allowed for the plaintiff to sue has passed. Since the plaintiff has not sued within the prescribed time, he is prohibited from suing now. (See Statute of Limitations, p. 42.)

It is the experience and conviction of courts, judges, and lawyers that justice is best served in litigation controversies by a full disclosure by both sides of all facts in their possession in advance of trial. Courts do not sit to reward cleverness, surprises, or tactical genius. Rather, they are established to analyze a transaction or event in detail, to ascertain the truth, and to reach a fair decision based on all the facts. Therefore, rules are established to permit each side to discover facts known to the other side which bear on the case prior to trial. Courts may require a *deposition*. This is an oral examination answering all manner of questions relating to the transaction at issue. The questions and answers are recorded and transcribed, and thus the party has given his version of events under oath. Therefore, taking a deposition is an effective device in developing the full truth. It permits both sides to know what the witness's version of an event will be at the trial and provides an equal opportunity to find corroborating or contradictory evidence. Courts can subpoena all relevant records upon request of counsel or on their own initiative.

Witness's Function   Witnesses testify to what they saw and heard or what they know about the matters at issue. They are subject to cross-examination by opposing counsel. There are rules of evidence to prevent anything being presented that is not relevant or authenticated. Hence, hearsay evidence is not admissible and documents must be identified as genuine before they are admitted into evidence to the

Allegations: charges

judge and jury. All witnesses' testimony is recorded by a court reporter during the trial. Not only witnesses' answers but also their demeanor and attitude are appraised by opposing counsel, the judge, and jury.

A witness should be careful not to display a bias or prejudice which could later impeach his credibility; for example, making disparaging remarks about the other workers. The witness should avoid showing resentment of questions and he should display candor and humility, even when the question seems to be irrelevant to the issues involved.

Anything doubtful or ambiguous in the testimony will be carefully probed. A witness should listen to the question and answer only as much as the question specifically requires. A witness is under oath and must tell the truth as he perceives it, or be guilty of *perjury*. Some attorneys say there is only one crime in court and that is to lie under oath. Perjury is held as the unforgivable crime. The outcome of the case obviously depends on the testimony of all the witnesses. Generally, the final decision comes down to credibility. What and whom does the jury believe based on the evidence presented?

Weight of Evidence

Generally, a fact may be proved directly or circumstantially. Direct proof is normally based on actual observation of witnesses. The reasoning process followed in the use of circumstantial evidence is that the existence of one or more known facts increases the probability that another fact is true. The accumulation of facts presented by exhibits and witnesses' testimony serves to arrive at truth.

In a civil case, the plaintiff must have a *preponderance* of the evidence in his favor to prove his case and have the judge and jury rule in his favor. In a criminal case, the state must prove its case beyond a *reasonable doubt* and with a moral certainty in order to find the defendant guilty. This is much stronger proof than is necessary in a civil tort action case.

The judge explains the law to the jury. He does this in the form of instructions by citing the law applicable in the case before

Deposition: testimony of a witness not in open court reduced to writing properly authenticated to be used at the trial

Preponderance: greater weight of evidence, or evidence which is more credible and convincing to the mind

Reasonable doubt: ordinary or usual knowledge of facts of a character calculated to induce a doubt in the mind of an ordinary intelligent and prudent businessman

them. He tells the jury what the law requires by way of factual elements so the jury may render a verdict for either the plaintiff or the defendant based on the facts as they determine them to be and the law as they apply it to those facts.

Jury Function   In a case of negligence or breach of duty, a jury has a two-step analysis to make. It must determine what the actual conduct of the plaintiff and the defendant was in fact, and it must determine whether such conduct was negligent. Once the conclusion of facts is made, then the jury must determine if conduct was negligent based on that same set of facts.

If the jury finds there has been *liability* on the part of the defendant, the jury must determine the amount of money to be given to the plaintiff to compensate him for his monetary losses and pain and suffering. The plaintiff is entitled to be reimbursed for his medical expenses. He is entitled to the full amount in money damages of any economic loss both present and in the future as a result of the defendant's negligence. The plaintiff is allowed monetary compensation for his pain and suffering also.

The plaintiff is indemnified or "made whole again."

Right of Appeal   A party against whom an adverse decision is rendered may wish to appeal to a higher court. An appellate appeal court does not re-try a case and hear all the evidence again. The appellate court considers primarily errors of law. The basic distinction is that an appellate court generally sits to review the question of law, and not the question of fact. It must be emphasized that an appeal will not overturn findings of fact made by a judge or jury, based on evaluation of all the testimony and evidence, unless the findings are clearly erroneous.

DOCTRINES AND PRINCIPLES OF LAW

Legal Expectations

What does the law expect of you with regard to your health care responsibilities? Health care practitioners seem to panic when this

Appellate court: that court where judgments of trial courts are reviewed or appealed
Liability: Responsibility for conduct falling below a certain standard which is the causal connection of the plaintiff's injury

question is raised, yet there is nothing mystical about what the law requires. Quite simply, *the law expects that you will provide safe facilities and quality care to patients and that you will maintain a standard of care equivalent to that of other hospitals in similar circumstances.* Above all, the law expects that you will at least do the patient no harm if you cannot do the patient any good. Thus, the law does not really expect too much, only that health practitioners act reasonably, and in accordance with professional standards.

The public's attitude toward health professionals has changed considerably in recent years. As the public has become more sophisticated, its attitude has shifted from one of great respect and near reverence for those engaged in the healing arts to a more realistic view that they are fallible human beings who should be held legally responsible for their actions like all other humans. "Medical mystique" can no longer protect doctors, nurses, and hospital personnel from being legally accountable for their actions.

Everyone must have some understanding of the basic principles of law, at least the simpler aspects of it. The law helps to settle disputes, improve society, and give redress for wrongs committed against persons in society. Many of us are not aware of how the many facets of the law affect our daily lives.

Legal System Is Dynamic   The legal system is not static. Rather, it is dynamic and constantly changing. It varies from locale to locale, and from one part of the country to another. The legal principles and doctrines which are applied to medical malpractice cases have evolved over many years, and courts are reluctant to reverse or modify these principles. However, technological and sociological changes, new medical practices, legislative enactments or reinterpretations of statutes and doctrines have changed the results obtained by applying these principles.

Statutory enactments are often far behind active practice in the health field. The legal process moves slowly to change existing standards because the law adheres to tradition and is reluctant to accept innovation. It is after society pressures for change that legislation is enacted. The statutory laws enacted by our representatives are the result of the majority of society's wishes. Abortions which were considered criminal, with some exceptions, a few decades ago are routine procedures today. This clearly indicates the response legislators have to changing attitudes in society. This type of reaction is

Raison d'etre: reason for being

presently being felt in the right to die with dignity isues. (See Part 2, p. 81.) Often health practitioners ask, "What is the law regarding such an issue?" They want specific answers, but it is not that easy. For example, look at the area of physician's asistants, or nurse practitioners. These job functions have existed for several years without any absolute guidelines or laws regarding specific acts. It is only within recent years that regulations were enacted in many states establishing various measurable criteria for physicians' asistants and nurse practitioners. What the law means will be established only after interpretation by the courts, either through litigation or other judicial process. The law is what the courts say it is, not what one thinks it is when reading the related statutory law of the state.

Malpractice and Safe Practice   If malpractice claims arose solely from errors in practice, it would be simple to prevent such claims. The health practitioner would simply render the best possible health care as consistently as possible. But malpractice suits also arise from other causes, including sociological and psychological causes.

The concept of malpractice claims prevention; it implies that affirmative steps be taken to prevent these claims from arising. There is a direct relationship between improved patient care and malpractice claims prevention.

Perhaps one of the contributing sociological reasons to why malpractice suits are becoming more frequent is the public's growing interest in medicine and awareness of medical facts. Discussions of medical topics appear daily in family magazines. Television programs dealing with medical subjects have likewise educated the public in many areas of medical practice.

Safe practice means performing the particular service or procedure for a patient in a competent manner. It means the nurse possesses the particular knowledge and skill necesary to perform the health care act he/she is engaged in with the same degree of knowledge and skill other nurses ordinarily possess and utilize when doing the same act. For example, a nurse who gives a patient medication by intramuscular injection is expected to know the human anatomy involved, the pharmacological and physiological effects of the drug, the indications of an undesirable response, and similar information. Safe practice and competent practice are fairly synonomous terms.

Reasonableness   Health practitioners are required to exercise ordinary or reasonable care to safeguard and protect the patient from any known or reasonably foreseeable harm. The courts have held this to be as much their responsibility as that of the physician. Many of the routine patient care activities involve the safety and security of the patient. The health practitioner is therefore expected to perform these acts without any special medical order or supervision. The kind and degree of health care necessary to protect a patient from harm will always depend on the particular circumstances of the case. The prime factor governing the type of care needed is the patient's physical and mental capacity to contribute to his own safety and security. In order to meet the legal responsibility to the patient, the health practitioner who is directed to carry out a medical act must understand both the execution of the medical procedure in question and its effect on the patient.

The fundamental guiding principle in health practice is that which a reasonably prudent person would do in the same situation. Along with this principle, one can consider custom and usage in the community, joint accreditation requirements, hospital policy, state licensing standards, and job descriptions.

For example, in the landmark decision of *Darling v. Charleston Community Hospital* (211 N.E. 2nd 53, Ill., 1965), the trial court allowed the Illinois Department of Public Health rules and regulations, the Charleston Community Hospital's bylaws, rules and regulations, and the Joint Commission on Accreditation's Standards for Hospital Accreditation to be admitted as documentary evidence. This permitted the jury to utilize these documents in determining the standard of care the hospital and staff were to meet in caring for patients. The court in fact found that the hospital failed to have a sufficient number of professional nurses trained to recognize the symptoms of a progressive gangrenous condition of a patient's fractured leg in a cast. The court also found that the physician in charge failed to get an orthopedic consultation as required by the medical staff bylaws. Not every unfavorable medical event is preventable, nor is every such event automatically the basis for a malpractice suit. No one expects the hospital or its staff to be "guarantors" of good health. This would be an unrealistic and unreasonable expectation. Instead, the hospital and its staff manifest that they are practitioners of competent and safe health care. In offering the public the means to good health care they imply they will not be negligent in the delivery of that same care.

Legislative Lag It is this combination of circumstances which dictate what a health professional's license permits one to do and what an employer expects the person to do. One can readily see that the two can often differ. Another point to consider is that the law itself generally follows actual practice. That is, the "custom and usage" community standards may permit a certain act, such as nurses starting intravenous fluids or removing surgical sutures, before legislation has been passed regulating the act. Innovation of specific approved medical-legal procedures is a slow process. It is hard to believe that there was a time when only a physician could take a blood pressure or give an injection. These were considered acts of medical practice and anyone performing these acts without a license was guilty of a criminal act; that is, practicing medicine without a license. Today laymen can perform either or both acts in appropriate circumstances.

The law is not the biblical equal of the Ten Commandments carved in stone. It is made by society for society, therefore, it follows logically that the law must change to meet the needs of the particular society for which it is structured.

Principles which are defined as fundamental truths or basic doctrines can be consistently applied to health care situations. But the outcome of the application of these principles can be and sometimes appears to be consistently inconsistent, which is the main concept to be understood. In any medico-legal situation that one will face, one can anticipate having to make judgments. The principle to be followed will be available, but one must select it appropriately to the set of circumstances one encounters.

Specific Doctrines and Principles of Law

The legal responsibility of the health practitioner is to be a practitioner of safe care. The various legal doctrines will give one insight into the ways in which the law fixes liability for acts of malpractice and will show how one may be subjected to a greater exposure of liability based upon various factors, or principles of law, or legal status of one's employer or your employment.

Doctrine of Personal Liability

If there is one rule that all should know and clearly understand, it is the fundamental rule of law that every person is liable for his own negligent conduct. This is known as the *rule of personal liability*. What this means is that the law does not permit a wrongdoer (in the tort-liability sense) to avoid legal liability for his own wrongdoing

Landmark decision: case or decision which establishes a new precedent of law for similar cases

even though someon else may also be sued and held legally liable for the wrongful conduct in question under another rule of law; it will not negate one's own responsibility.

For example, a doctor tells a nurse to execute a medical order which both know to be improper and says he will take full responsibility for any harmful consequences. If the nurse proceeds and the patient is injured, both will be held liable. The doctor's assurance would not help the nurse to avoid personal liability. This occurs in an operating room situation where the sponge count is not correct when the operation is concluded. The operating surgeon tells the nurses assisting him that he thinks all the sponges are out of the operative site and he is going to close the incision. Hospital policy states the sponge count must be verified before and after the surgical procedure. If the count is not verified and the patient is injured because of a sponge left in the patient, the nurse would be personally liable for her/his own negligence in not making certain the count was correct. The fact that she/he was following the surgeon's instructions would make the surgeon liable also, but would not be a defense for her own negligence.

Or, a registered nurse directs a licensed practical nurse to perform a nursing function which the latter is not qualified to carry out. Assume that the licensed practical nurse follows the order without question and harm occurs to the patient and assume that the registered nurse knows or should have known the licensed practical nurse is not qualified. In this event, if the registered nurse is found liable, would the licensed practical nurse be relieved of liability? The answer is no. And the converse is true. The licensed practical nurse, or anyone else, should know his or her own qualifications and limitations. The licensed practical nurse would be personally liable for performing an act which injures a patient and for which she is not qualified. The registered nurse would be liable for assigning the function to the licensed practical nurse when the registered nurse knows the nursing function is one which a licensed practical nurse is not normally qualified to perform.

However, assume the registered nurse gives the licensed practical nurse a routine nursing assignment, which as a licensed practical nurse she ordinarily would be able to perform without difficulty. For example, the licensed practical nurse is assigned to give medications to the patients. While giving medications, the licensed practical nurse gives a patient the wrong dosage and the patient is injured. The licensed practical nurse has been negligent and this negligence, giving the wrong medication, caused the patient to be injured. Where does liability rest in this case? In this set of facts, only the licensed practical nurse would be held liable for negligence in carrying out an assignment clearly within her capabilities. The registered nurse has a right to expect the licensed practical nurse to be capable of performing functions carried out by similarly prepared licensed practical nurses, unless the registered nurse has been notified of a limitation placed on the licensed practical nurse. It is the duty of the nursing service department to thoroughly check the credentials and qualifications of its employees before assigning them staff duties. The registered nurse has a right to assume her co-workers are competent unless put on notice to the contrary.

Doctrine of Respondeat Superior

Another related legal doctrine which has a significant effect upon the health practitioner's legal liability is the *doctrine of respondeat superior,* "let the master respond." The doctrine of respondeat superior is a legal doctrine which holds an employer liable for the negligent acts of his employees which occur while they are carrying out his orders or otherwise serving his interests. Since most health practitioners are employed by others, this doctrine is of paramount importance. The legal effect of the doctrine of respondeat superior is that it creates liability on the part of an employer for the negligent acts of his employees. The doctrine of respondeat superior applies only when there is an employer-employee relationship and only with respect to negligent acts committed within the scope of that employment. The theory behind the doctrine is that one who is an employer should be held legally responsible for the conduct of those employees whose actions he is obligated to direct or control. Often the critical test in determining liability is who had control over the employee. For example, Dolores Darner, R.N., works in the out patient department at Healing Arts Hospital giving injections to patients everyday. At a certain time on a particular day, Dolores gives an injection and injuries a patient's arm, and paralysis results. Who is liable? Both Dolores Darner and the employer, Healing Arts Hospital, may be held liable if Dolores was a bonafide employee and was doing work assigned by the hospital as a proper function for which she is qualified. The hospital or employer is liable for all the negligent acts committed by the nurse that are related to the function of the nurse in the service of the employer.

But suppose however, a neighbor asks Dolores Darner, R.N., to give insulin to her mother in her home. If injury results in this situation, such as footdrop or arm injury, who would be liable? Obviously,

Dolores Darner, R.N., alone. Why? Dolores Darner was not functioning as an employee within the scope of the out patient department, her job description, or the policies or procedures of Healing Arts Hospital. At the time she undertook to administer the injection, Dolores may have been a bona fide employee of the hospital but she was never assigned the function of giving non-hospital patients hypodermic injections. Dolores Darner was not functioning within the scope of her authority. (See Appendix IV.) Therefore, one element is missing and the Healing Arts Hospital would not be held liable. Only Dolores Darner would be responsible and liable.

Consider the case where an employee at the hospital asks Dolores Darner, R.N., to give her mother an insulin injection in the home. Suppose Dolores is cautious, sophisticated, and astute. In order to be certain she was operating properly, let us assume Dolores Darner, R.N., asks the Director of Nursing, Ms. Kay Lily, R.N., if she may give injections of insulin to the employee's mother. Assume that Ms. Kay Lily gives permission to Dolores Darner to administer the insulin injections to the employee's mother. If the mother is injured from the insulin injections, who would be liable now? The answer is that both Kay Lily, the Director of Nurses, and Dolores Darner giving the injections would be liable, but not under the doctrine of respondeat superior. The elements for applying the doctrine of respondeat superior are missing. There is no employer–employee relationship in this set of facts. Also, both nurses were functioning out of the scope of their authority. Each of the actors or nurses involved are liable under the doctrine of personal liability. The Director of Nurses had no authority to authorize Dolores Darner, R.N., to give insulin injections to persons in the home, unless there was something specific in the hospital's charter and bylaws regarding a home nursing care program. Without this authority Kay Lily, the Director of Nurses, would be liable under the doctrine of personal liability. Dolores Darner would be liable for her own negligence and since Kay Lily could not delegate authority she did not have, Healing Arts Hospital would not be held liable under these circumstances.

Indemnification Even though the doctrine of respondeat superior provides the injured patient with another party to sue, it does not relieve the negligent practitioner of his own liability. If the employer is otherwise blameless for the negligent conduct of a health practitioner employee, the employer might be obligated under respondeat superior to pay damages to the injured patient. The employer may recover the amount of damages paid in a separate action. It is the employer's right to be indemnified. The critical factor to determine liability under this doctrine is to decide who had the legal right to direct and control the employee's activities at the time the negligent act was committed. This factor allows more individuals or corporations to be sued and increases the chances for recovery for the plaintiff. It also means the hospital could institute a separate suit against the health practitioner to recover the money paid by the employer for vicarious liability. For example, a health care practitioner gives an injection to a patient causing partial paralysis of the left leg. The patient sues the employer hospital and the court awards thirty thousand dollars ($30,000) as compensatory damages for the hospital's liability. The hospital has a right to sue the health care practitioner for $30,000 because of the health care practitioner's negligence which caused the employer to suffer a loss and for which the employer has a right at law to be made whole again or indemnified.

If a patient were to be injured by a nurse's aide who had a limited income and many financial obligations, it would mean that the patient's chance to recover monetary damages would be negligible under the doctrine of personal liability. Therefore, by utilizing the appropriate doctrine, such as respondeat superior, recovery may be obtained from the employer to prevent an innocent victim, the patient, from being injured without any available recovery under the law. This type of sanction encourages the employer to employ competent personnel to reduce legal risk.

Doctrine of Borrowed Servant

The *borrowed servant doctrine* is usually considered when discussing the respondeat superior principle. In the borrowed servant doctrine, as the name implies, the employee is "borrowed" for a particular purpose or agency. The classical example occurs in the operating room. Although the scrub nurse or operating room technician is an employee of the hospital, he is paid and controlled by the administration of the hospital for the purpose of a specific operation. But that same employee is directed or controlled by the surgeon during the operation; therefore, depending on the facts of the case, the negligent liability of the scrub technician may vicariously involve the surgeon performing the operation rather than the hospital which employs the technician. Here the law infers that the one directing or

Indemnified: made whole again, reimbursed
Vicarious: substitute

controlling the actions of the employee has the greater responsibility over the one who merely pays the employee. For example, the scrub technician is asked for a surgical count of sponges at the end of an operative procedure. Assume that the surgeon has control and directs the count of the sponges and makes the final decision regarding the accuracy of the count. If the count is wrong and a sponge is left in the patient, both the scrub technician and the doctor would be liable. You may hear this referred to as the "captain of the ship doctrine" also. Its meaning again is obvious. The captain of a ship has traditionally been held responsible for all those under his supervision. Similarly, the surgeon who controls the actions of the assisting doctors, anesthetist, and the technicians is considered the "captain of the ship" in the operating room. The surgeon has control over all the members of the operating team. He makes the final decision.

The courts have ruled both that the hospital has been responsible and that it has not been responsible in cases where sponges have been left inside patients. The courts have also held physicians responsible in some cases and not responsible in others. On analyzing these cases where the parties have been held responsible, it was found the liable parties generally had "control" over the sponge count or were completely responsible for it.

For example, in the cases where hospital policy clearly stated the sponge count was to be taken before and after surgery and verified by the circulating nurse, the hospital was held liable when sponges were left inside the patient. The court reasoned the hospital, through its employees, was in control of the sponge count. In the cases where the operating surgeon had the final responsibility to decide all sponges were out of the operative site, the operating surgeon was held liable if a sponge remained in the patient. The court reasoned the operating surgeon was in control of the sponge count and therefore responsible.

New Kinds of "Employees"   There is a new area of relationships developing in hospitals. Doctors are forming corporations. In many states by recent statute, professional persons such as doctors and lawyers may form corporations. The general rule of law is that the corporation is solely liable for any negligence resulting from members of the corporation. This is not generally true for physicians in professional corporations. They may also be held liable individually, or personally. Several hospitals have contracted certain areas of service, such as the emergency room or out patient department, to individual physicians or to a group of physicians practicing as a corporation, or independent contractors. In some instances, the hospitals pay directly the individual physician and corporation. In other instances, the patient is billed directly and the hospital does not act as agent for collection of the fees. There are all types of modifications of services between the patient, the doctor, and the hospital. In the event of negligence, who is liable? It is evident that many factors must be analyzed in each case to determine who will be held responsible. The entire economic structure of health care will play a prime role in future malpractice suits in determining who should and who is most able to bear the economic burden of financing legal redress for the patient.

No-Fault Trend   As a corrollary, there is a trend to develop no-fault insurance for malpractice claims comparable to the no-fault insurance for automobile claims recently enacted by several state legislatures. The thought is to include a cost or premium for no-fault insurance in one's health insurance plan. In the event that someone is injured in a hospital or health-related agency, there would be no necessity to have any litigation to determine who was the cause of the injury or to determine who was at fault. Instead, there would be a procedure to ascertain the amount of damages incurred by the patient. This could be done by one or two physicians, a committee or board of doctors, lawyers and laymen, or a board of review. Once the damages were reasonably ascertained, they would be paid. Naturally, there are proponents and opponents of the trend. At the present time this innovative doctrine has not been accepted but it is still discussed as a viable alternative.

Doctrine of the Reasonably Prudent Man

If there is such a thing as the most important principle or doctrine in medical-legal law, it is the *reasonably prudent man theory*. This is the standard requiring an individual to perform a function as any reasonable man of ordinary prudence, with comparable education, skills, and training under similar circumstances would perform that same function. It has been described as requiring a person of ordinary sense to use ordinary care and skill. Health care practitioners are required to act as similar health care practitioners would in similar circumstances. Although a simple concept, it is difficult to give a set of definite rules that would guarantee one would not be found negligent or liable if these rules were followed. Everything is relative to the particular set of circumstances at a particular time. The health care practitioner should remember that one is not judged by the standard expected of the brightest or the least bright health practitioner. He is not judged by what he should have done after reviewing a particular act in hindsight. He is judged on what the average reasonably prudent health practitioner is expected to do faced with a certain set of facts and circumstances and not what one would do two weeks later or after several hours of reflection. The standard is what the reasonably prudent practitioner would be expected to do now, at the particular time, and under the immediate particular circumstances. Reduced to the bare essentials, one is expected to demonstrate the skill, judgment, and quality of care common to the profession in any hospital, agency, or locale.

Application of Reasonably Prudent Man Doctrine   In order to appreciate the application of the principle of a factual situation, two cases are presented for comparison. In the first case, Laura Newhall [1] was admitted to Central Hospital with a diagnosis of bursitis in her right knee. On the second day following admission to the hospital, she put on her call bell. Laura Newhall testified she waited for "a long time." Because there was no response to her call for help, she proceeded to get out of bed to go to the lavatory. While attempting to do this she slipped and fell and said she injured her back.

What, if any, liabilities do you think were determined by the court under these circumstances?

Some arguments that might be made for the hospital were that it was not "a long time" for the patient to have waited. This, of course, is a question of fact for the jury to determine based on the evidence. If the nurses were engaged in other critical activities, such as an emergency, they could not be reasonably expected to be in two places at one time and this would be a good defense. However, that was not the case. The argument of short staffing on the unit would also not justify the lack of response.

The patient argued that she was essentially immobile because of the bursitis. Any reasonably prudent nurse could foresee that a patient with such a diagnosis needed attention to basic bodily needs. It was also foreseeable that a patient under these circumstances not getting a response to her call within a reasonable time could fall while trying to go to the lavatory.

The verdict was $30,594 against the hospital. The court said in its opinion that attempting to leave the bed when no bed pan was

[1]   *Newhall v. Central Vermont Hospital*, 349 A 2d 890 (Vt. 1975).

available was not the only course of action that could be taken. But it is certainly the one most reasonably to be expected from the average patient.

The outcome varied in a somewhat similar sets of facts. Mrs. Celia Minks was admitted to the McDowell Hospital [2] for a diagnostic workup. The evening of her admission she was being routinely prepared for a barium enema x-ray. As part of the preparations, the patient had ordered and was given a routine sleeping medication (carbital grains 1½ for sleep). In the middle of the night the patient awakened, got out of bed and proceeded down a hallway to the bathroom. The patient fell down a flight of stairs fracturing both of her legs. The patient sued the nurses on duty and the hospital. Who, if anyone, would be liable as determined by the court under these circumstances?

The court ruled in favor of the nurses and the hospital. The hospital staff had acted reasonably under the circumstances. There was no indication from any actions on the part of Celia Minks to put the staff on notice that Mrs. Minks might be disoriented or confused or would react any differently than the average patient. The patient is entitled to that care which his age, mental and physical condition warrant as necessary for his safety. The very young, elderly, or handicapped patients require a higher duty of care than other patients. The hospital is not an insurer or guarantor of the health and safety of all patients. The staff met its obligation by giving reasonable care under the circumstances. The issue of contributory negligence might also be raised. Everyone, including patients, is required to act as a reasonably prudent person under the particular circumstances. There may be a question whether Mrs. Minks' actions met the standard of a reasonably prudent patient. In states that recognize the doctrine of contributory negligence, it is a defense to the charge of negligence. This means that a plaintiff who had contributed to this own injury no matter how slightly could not recover for his injuries.

These two cases serve to illustrate how the courts look at all the evidence presented and apply the standard of reasonableness to those circumstances. Did the defendant act as a reasonably prudent nurse or health care practitioner would have in these set of circumstances? The determination of a defendant's negligence and liability will depend on the outcome of measuring the defendant's actions against the standard of the actions expected of a reasonably prudent nurse in similar circumstances at a similar time. If the actions of the defendant

[2] *McDowell Hospital v. Minks,* 529 So. 2d 360 (Kentucky, 1975).

fall below this standard of reasonable action, the defendant will be found liable for negligent action.

Doctrine of Corporate Negligence

Corporate negligence means that the hospital or health care agency as an entity is negligent. Those entrusted with the task of providing proper facilities fail to carry out the corporation's purpose. It is the failure of the corporation to follow an established standard of conduct to which all health care corporations should conform in a given situation.

The doctrine of corporate negligence or liability, as a doctrine of law applied to hospitals, is relatively new. The determination of negligence is based on violation or breach of the duty owed to the patient by the hospital or health center. The landmark case of *Darling v. Charleston Community Memorial Hospital,* decided in 1965 by the Supreme Court of Illinois, was the beginning of the legal clarification of the roles and responsibilities of the hospital trustees. It stated that the hospital does not consist of two organizations, business and medical, but rather that it is a single organization for which the board of trustees is ultimately responsible.

In the famous landmark decision of the *Darling v. Charleston Community Hospital,*[3] the facts of the case briefly are as follows:

Darling, the plaintiff, was an 18-year-old college student who played on the football team. Darling was injured while playing football and was taken to the emergency room of Charleston Community Hospital. The doctor on emergency room call on that particular day was a general practitioner. The physician took x-rays, diagnosed fractures of both bones below the knee in the right leg. He then reduced the fracture and applied a cast to the leg.

Darling complained of pain continuously. Three days after applying the cast, the general practitioner split the cast. Darling continued to complain of pain. There was evidence that circulation was impaired and there was a foul odor at the area of the fracture. There were no orthopedic specialists or consultations of any kind. Approximately two weeks later Darling was transferred to another hospital and given the care of an orthopedic surgeon, but it was too late. The leg had to be amputated.

The most important issue decided in the case was the standard of care for determining hospital liability. The court found the hospital

3 *Darling v. Charleston Community Hospital,* 211 N.E. 2d 53 (Illinois, 1965).

failed to meet the standard of care due to Darling because neither consultation nor examination by skilled orthopedic surgeons were utilized and there were insufficient trained nurses capable of recognizing the progressive gangrenous condition which resulted in an amputation.

The court allowed the rules and regulations of the Illinois Department of Health, the hospital licensing act, the standards of the Joint Commission on Accreditation of Hospitals, and the bylaws, rules and regulations of Charleston Hospital to be introduced into evidence.

The verdict against the hospital was $110,000. The physician had settled prior to trial for $40,000. The hospital was found liable under the doctrine of corporate negligence. This means the hospital as an entity is negligent. The hospital has the obligation of giving due care to every patient utilizing its facilities. The hospital had failed to meet the established standard of care in this situation. In its opinion, the court said, "the governing body of each hospital shall be responsible for the operation of the hospital, for the selection of medical staff, and for the quality of care rendered in the hospital."

The governing body of the hospital or health center is the board of trustees. Case law, statutes, and standards of accreditation all recognize the ultimate, non-delegable corporate and legal responsibility of the board to assure that quality care is provided. Vesting of the legal responsibility for patient care is more clearly recognized and understood today than ever before. Each judicial decision reaffirms the fact that the governing boards of hospitals and health care centers have the ultimate responsibility for the operation and function of the agency for providing proper patient care.

The board is charged with the right and the duty to monitor the quality of health care being provided by the professional staff. It has the final authority to satisfy the corporate objectives. All others, administrator, medical staff, and comptroller, have delegated authority to act within defined parameters of operations. The actual monitoring should be delegated to the medical staff because they, by professional training and experience, are most capable of performing this important task. Generally, board members are not "health experts." They are not expected to do the actual monitoring, but they should have sufficient expertise to be able to approve the appointment of a professional staff that will be accountable for its share of the function of quality control. The board members must carefully scrutinize the reports submitted by the professional staff, and must assure themselves that there is continuous review, analysis, and evaluation of patient care. Concomitantly, recommendations by the medical staff should be acted on and communicated to the staff. Facts and documented objective information should support recommendations for appointments, denial of privileges, and changes in policy. No action should be taken unless convinced by objective data that the action will serve the best interest of both the patient and the institution. Failure of the hospital and the board members to meet their obligation to the patient could result in liability.

In California in 1974, Dr. Nork,[4] an orthopedist, was found negligent in his care of at least 30 patients. The verdict was $3,710,447 of which $2,000,000 constituted *punitive damages* because of Dr. Nork's wanton reckless disregard of the patients in his care.

The evidence in the case showed that the hospital, the medical staff, and the staff licensing board never took any action against Dr. Nork although it knew or should have known he was causing injury to his patients.

The main case against Dr. Nork was that brought by Albert Gonzales. The facts briefly were that Albert Gonzales was examined by Dr. Nork in November 1967 for back pain. Dr. Nork's diagnosis was acute disc herniation. A lumbar myelogram was done; it was within normal limits. In spite of this and without consultation, Dr. Nork did a laminectomy and spinal fusion on Mr. Gonzales. Albert Gonzales complained of pain immediately after surgery in his back, legs and right thigh. There were conflicting notations in Gonzales' medical record. A November 30 note by Dr. Nork said he "had done extremely well, no complaints." The nurse's note of the same date stated "ambulated with help for ten minutes, had to be helped to the bathroom, complains of terrible pain and right leg felt paralyzed." Gonzales became progressively worse and by November 12, 1970, he was considered to be permanently disabled.

Mercy Hospital where Gonzales was a patient was also found liable for negligence under the doctrine of corporate negligence. The court held that the hospital owed the patient a duty of care which included protecting the patient from acts of medical negligence by the hospital's staff physician. The words used were, "If the hospital knows, or has reason to know, or should have known such acts were likely to occur." The court held the hospital was corporately responsible for the conduct of the medical staff.

The courts expect hospitals to have policies and procedures to

Punitive damages: money awarded as a penalty; damages relating to punishment

4   *Gonzales v. Nork.*

reasonably assure proper patient care and to take appropriate action against those who do not comply. Anything less is not acceptable.

Doctrine of Res Ipsa Loquitur

The law expects that a plaintiff making certain charges or allegations of negligence against a defendant will be prepared to prove those charges by a preponderance of evidence. In general, the plaintiff must prove that the defendant did not meet a professional standard of conduct and that the plaintiff was injured as a result. There is a presumption at law that a nurse, physician, or any health care practitioner has met the professional standard of care he is practicing. It is up to the party alleging negligence to meet the burden of proving that the defendant (health care professional) has not met the standard. The presumption is somewhat akin to the individual charged with committing a crime. The alleged criminal comes into court presumed to be innocent. The state has the burden of proving beyond a reasonable doubt and with a moral certainty that the alleged criminal did in fact commit the acts with which he is charged. It is not up to the alleged criminal to prove he did not do it. The more difficult posture is the burden of proving something. Under certain circumstances and specifically under the res ipsa loquitur doctrine, the burden of proof shifts. If the plaintiff can establish the elements necessary for the application of res ipsa loquitur, then the defendant comes into court with the inference of having been negligent and must disprove it.

Elements of Res Ipsa Loquitur   *Res ipsa loquitur* means "the thing speaks for itself." It is self-evident. This doctrine has limited application, that is, not all states allow this doctrine to be applied in medical-legal cases. However, the doctrine is expanding in many states, such as California, Florida, Massachusetts, Minnesota, and others with or without qualifications. It is generally applied in situations where a patient was injured while unconscious. He had no way of knowing all the facts because of the unconsciousness and would probably not be able to establish negligence by a preponderance of evidence having to carry the burden of proof. The elements that the plaintiff must prove to utilize the doctrine are: 1) this type of injury does not normally occur unless there was negligence; 2) the injury was caused by an agency under the exclusive control of the defendant; and 3) the plaintiff did not contribute to his injury in any way.

Once these elements have been established, it is up to the defendant—nurse, physician, or other health care practitioner—to prove he was not negligent and did not cause the patient's injury. If the defendant fails in his burden of proof, the jury may draw the inference that the defendant has been negligent.

Purpose of Doctrine   The purpose of the application of the res ipsa loquitur doctrine is to equalize the parties in the case. Where the plaintiff has been injured but is at an unfair disadvantage, not of his own making, the doctrine assists the plaintiff. It does not, nor was it intended to, create evidence or encourage unwarranted litigation. The sole purpose of the doctrine was to reduce the plaintiff's handicap in proving his injury under certain selected circumstances. All elements of the doctrine must be met; if any element is missing, such as the injury occurred from an agency or instrumentality not in the defendant's control, the plaintiff cannot plead res ipsa loquitur.

Kinds of Cases Where Res Ipsa Loquitur Is Applicable   The classical application of this doctrine is the case where a sponge or instrument is left in the patient's operative site. Another is where the patient is operated on for a cholecystectomy or a hysterectomy or a hemorrhoidectomy and after the operation is unable to move his hand or arm because of injury to the ulnar or radial nerves from positioning during the operation. There are other cases where the wrong limb had been operated on or amputated.

Contemporary Case Applying Res Ipsa Loquitur Doctrine   Frank Shields [5] was a candidate for a kidney transplant. During the waiting period, Mr. Shields underwent hemodialysis on several occasions. The procedure was performed at the hospital with hospital equipment. The attending physician, Dr. King, was not an employee of the hospital but supervised the dialysis procedure.

Mr. Shields had a hemodialysis treatment on July 1, 1966. On July 5, 1966, another hemodialysis was done utilizing Mr. Shield's own blood for priming the machine. There was no indication of infection at any time. The patient, Frank Shields, went into severe shock shortly after the hemodialysis procedure. He died two days later from

Agency: includes every relation in which one person acts for or represents another by latter's authority

Directed verdict: evidence presented by plaintiff is insufficient to have to go to jury and case is dismissed

[5] *Shields v. King*, 317 N.E. 2d 922 (Ohio. App. 1973).

an escherica coli septicemia, contamination of the blood or the dialysis machine with escherica coli bacteria.

Trial court granted a directed verdict for the physician and hospital. The case was appealed and the appellate court held that the doctrine of res ipsa loquitur could be appropriately applied to this set of facts.

In applying the elements of the doctrine, this type of injury does not ordinarily occur unless there was negligence. The physician and hospital staff were jointly in exclusive control of the instrumentality causing the injury. The plaintiff did not contribute to the injury.

The court found that the inference to be reasonably drawn from the circumstances was that the defendants were negligent, and in order to be found not negligent the defendants should rebut and overcome the allegations made by the plaintiff.

Doctrine of Foreseeability

This is a principle of law that holds an individual liable for all the natural and proximate consequences of any negligent acts to another individual to whom a duty is owed, and which could or should have been reasonably foreseen under the circumstances. A simple definition is that an individual could reasonably foresee that certain action or inaction on his part could result in injury to another individual. It also means that the injury actually suffered must be related to the foreseeable injury.

The nurse or health care practitioner has special training and more education than the average layman. The standard refers to what reasonably prudent nurses would be expected to anticipate as potentially harmful to an individual. If other professional nurses could anticipate harm in a similar set of circumstances, the nurse involved is also expected to anticipate that harm.

A classical example is the medication nurse who finds that the physician has written a medication order without a route of administration. This is an incomplete order. If the nurse were to supply the route she thought the doctor intended and it was wrong, resulting in injury to the patient, the nurse would be liable. It would be clearly foreseeable that the nurse was taking a chance and harm could result. The nurse's duty would be to resolve the incomplete order and have the doctor specify the particular route of administration.

In a New York case,[6] a 23-year-old male medical student was

6 *Cohen v. New York,* 382 N.Y. S 2d. 128 (New York, 1975).

admitted to the psychiatric unit with the diagnosis of paranoid schizo-
phrenia. There was an admission note that said the patient had suicidal
tendencies. In spite of the diagnosis and admission note, the patient
was not restricted and was not placed on suicidal precautions. He was
allowed off the unit and then committed suicide. The personal representative of the estate sued and the court ruled in favor of the estate.
The court said it was reasonable to foresee that such a patient would
attempt suicide. Under the circumstances there was a duty to impose
restraint on the patient's freedom to protect the patient from injuring
himself. There have been unfortunate situations where patients have
committed suicide where it could not have been anticipated and therefore there was no liability. Another factor in the foreseeability doctrine
is that of notice. If the nurses or health care practitioners have never
been put on notice by any act of a patient, they cannot be reasonably
expected to know a patient has that propensity. On the other hand,
where a patient has attempted suicide unsuccessfully, the nurses then
are said "to know or should know" the patient will attempt suicide.
The act is then foreseeable and there is a duty to take appropriate
action to protect the patient.

Improvisation and Warranties   The doctrine of foreseeability is an
appropriate place to deal with warranties. A *warranty* is generally a
promise that the article or goods sold are reasonably fit for the general
purpose for which they were intended. The warranty is basically a
contract between the seller and the purchaser. Most equipment purchased in a hospital today has a warranty. The parties to the warranty
are expected to deal fairly with one another. Therefore, it is expected
that the equipment purchased by the hospital will be free from defects
and fit for the purpose for which it was purchased. The hospital pur-
chasing the equipment is expected to comply with the conditions set
forth in the warranty and to notify the vendor (seller) of any defect in
the equipment so the defects may be corrected.

Responsibility for Warranty   As more and more sophisticated equipment becomes part of the technological health care system, it is necessary to be aware of any warranties involved in equipment which you
may be using. In order for a warranty to stay in effect, all conditions
of the warranty must be performed. For example, if a particular piece
of equipment requires a special lubricant for functioning, then any
substitution could negate the warranty. If sterile distilled water is
required to be used in a particular piece of equipment, substitution of
tap water could foreseeably cause malfunctioning. If the malfunction-

ing occurred at a critical time and the patient was harmed as a result, the nurse would be liable and the manufacturer of the equipment would generally not be held liable under such circumstances.

Routine Equipment Check   It is a basic standard of hospital care that equipment used for and by patients should be safe and function properly. The hospital must have some type of system to routinely check equipment and supplies so that all are maintained in proper working order. It is evident that any reasonably prudent professional could foresee that harm could come to a patient if equipment is not checked appropriately. (For example, see Vignette 18.)

Case on Foreseeability   The Florida Court of Appeals [7] recently ruled in favor of the hospital and the emergency room personnel in a case involving the issue of foreseeability.

A patient, F. Clayton, was brought to the James Archer Smith Hospital emergency room by his grandmother. The grandmother told the emergency room nurse that her grandson had taken "acid." There was no apparent need for immediate emergency attention for F. Clayton. The grandmother was advised by the emergency room staff to take the grandson to Jackson Memorial Hospital because that hospital had testing facilities to determine what drugs were taken.

While the grandmother was transporting her grandson F. Clayton to Jackson Memorial Hospital he became very agitated. F. Clayton jumped from the grandmother's car, ran into a nearby apartment house and stabbed Mr. E. Nance to death.

The widow of E. Nance sued the emergency room personnel of James Archer Smith Hospital and the hospital. Mrs. Nance charged the defendants with negligence. She alleged the defendants knew or should have known that F. Clayton was a danger to himself and to others and therefore were responsible for the stabbing death of her husband.

The trial court rejected the arguments of the widow, M. Nance. The court said there was no demonstrable evidence that the defendants could have reasonably anticipated the homicidal act of F. Clayton. While F. Clayton was in the emergency room he did not act in such a bizarre manner that would cause the defendants to foresee that he would act in such a way as to cause the death of E. Nance.

[7]   *Nance v. James Archer Smith Hospital, Inc.,* 329 So. 2d 277 (Fla. App. 1976).

Doctrine of Outrageous Conduct
or *Tort of Emotional Distress*

This is a relatively new and evolving principle of law. The doctrine of outrageous conduct allows a plaintiff to base his cause of action on intentional or negligent emotional distress caused by the defendant's action.

The judicial system has been cautious in allowing cases to be brought and verdicts to be given where the cause of action alleged is an emotional injury without any discernible accompanying physical injury.

Normally, anyone alleging negligence on the part of a defendant would have to establish that there was a duty owed to the plaintiff, that the duty was breached and the plaintiff suffered tangible physical damages proximately caused by the defendant. However, in an Iowa [8] case the Supreme Court of that state recognized the elements of outrageous conduct to be: 1) outrageous conduct by the defendant; 2) intentionally causing or by reckless disregard of the probability of causing, the defendant causes emotional distress to the plaintiff; 3) the plaintiff suffers severe or extreme emotional distress; and 4) the actual and proximate causation of the emotional distress was the defendant's outrageous conduct.

In the Iowa case, the funeral director mislead the plaintiff regarding the entire funeral of his father and stepmother killed in an automobile accident. The funeral director told the plaintiff it was necessary to have sealed caskets because of the odor and conditions of the bodies. The funeral director made these and other false statements to the plaintiff causing the plaintiff severe emotional distress.

The Restatement of Torts [9] defines outrageous conduct as that conduct which is "beyond all possible bounds of decency, and to be regarded as atrocious and utterly intolerable in a civilized community."

The case of *Johnson v. Woman's Hospital* [10] shocked the sensitivities of the court. The facts in the case were as follows:

Mrs. Johnson gave premature birth to a stillborn child. She was very upset. She spoke with a nurse on the floor about burial of the infant. It was Mrs. Johnson's understanding that the hospital would bury the infant in accord with the usual traditions of human dignity.

8   *Meyer v. Nottger,* 241 N.W. 2d 911 (Iowa, 1976).
9   *Restatement of Torts* (2d Edition), Section 46 (1965).
10 *Johnson v. Woman's Hospital,* 527 S.W. 133 (Tenn. App. 1975).

Approximately six weeks postpartum, Mrs. Johnson had access to a pathologist's report regarding her delivery. Upon reading the report, Mrs. Johnson became concerned about the disposition of her baby's body. She returned to Woman's Hospital where she had originally delivered the infant. One of the nurse's employed at the hospital handed Mrs. Johnson a gallon container with the shrivelled body of her baby floating in formaldehyde. The court was outraged at the unconscionable conduct on the part of the hospital and its employees. The court awarded the Johnson parents $100,000 recovery against the hospital under the doctrine of outrageous conduct for the emotional distress inflicted on the Johnsons'.

There are antagonists to the expansion of this doctrine of outrageous conduct by the courts. They argue it would mean potential liability for any type of mental or emotional distress and that the courts will be inundated with fraudulent and frivolous claims. The counterargument is that the jury system is capable of discerning legitimate claims from illegitimate claims lacking merit. The courts are recognizing and deciding accordingly that an individual who has been subjected to emotional distress by an individual who could reasonably know that the natural and probable consequences of the action would cause mental anguish to the other individual has a right to redress in the courts. The courts are as capable of weighing the evidence and reaching an equitable and just decision in these cases as well as in cases where there are tangible injuries. Finally, no one should be denied his right of redress under the law where the claim is meritorious.

DEFENSES AND DAMAGES

There are certain defenses to the charge of negligence that may be utilized by the defendant in preparing his case against the plaintiff. Some issues raised by the defendant will serve to mitigate or alleviate the charges or damages in certain cases. Other defenses may serve to have the charges dismissed or to completely prohibit the plaintiff from recovery against the defendant. Some of the more common defenses will be dealt with in this chapter. The types of redress and damages the plaintiff may be entitled to are also explained.

Redress: satisfaction for the injury sustained

Contributory Negligence

Contributory negligence is an affirmative defense. This means the defendant must raise the issue and establish by evidence that the patient was guilty of contributory negligence. Every individual is expected to act with ordinary care. That is, every individual is held to the standard of acting as a reasonably prudent individual would act in the same set of circumstances. It is the duty and responsibility of every patient to use the same care and prudence that another individual in the same set of circumstances would use. Therefore, if the patient fails to act according to this standard and his action or inaction contributes to his injury, it can be a barrier to suing or to receiving any recovery from the hospital or health care practitioners. This doctrine is not recognized in all states, but where it is recognized it is a complete defense to the defendant once it has been established.

An example of the application of this doctrine is a typical hospital scene. The nurse is giving a postoperative cholecystectomy patient morning care. The patient is clear, lucid, and rational. It is a routine situation. The nurse tells the patient to rest following the bath and she will return to get him out of bed. She further tells the patient not to get out of bed by himself because he is weak from the operation and may fall. The nurse leaves the room. The patient decides to go to the bathroom by himself. The patient proceeds to get out of bed, slips and falls, and breaks a leg. Who is liable? The patient clearly did not act as a reasonably prudent patient. He was the cause of his own injury. The nurse was not negligent unless she knew or had reason to know the patient would attempt to get out of bed by himself. The patient would probably not have any legal recourse under this set of facts. (For example, see Vignette 30).

Comparative Negligence

There are some states which recognize the doctrine of comparative negligence. It is, as the term implies, a doctrine in which the negligence of the plaintiff and the defendant is compared. It is an apportionment of damages based on the acts the parties are found to have committed. There are degrees of failure to exercise due care. If the omission or failure to take due care in a certain situation is that which a reasonably prudent man takes in his own affairs, the individual is said to be ordinarily negligent. If there is an intentional failure to perform an obvious duty in reckless, willful, and wanton disregard of the consequences to the person or property of another, the individual is said to be grossly negligent. Many states are moving in the direction of recognizing the doctrine of comparative negligence. It is believed to be a more equitable doctrine than that of contributory negligence which prevents a plaintiff any redress even where a defendant has been grossly negligent. (For example, see Vignette 30.)

Statute of Limitations

Anyone who wishes to sue or seek redress for a possible injury must do so within a specified period of time set by law makers. An individual has from the time he knew or had reason to know he had a cause of action to a specified length of time to file suit. This is called the *statute of limitations.* If the plaintiff fails to file within this statutory time, he is barred from making a claim against the defendant or a recovery. This is important. Regardless of how valid a plaintiff's case may be based on the merits, the case will be lost procedurally if the plaintiff fails to make a timely filing of his cause. The passing of time makes the gathering of facts difficult. A potential defendant should have the opportunity to defend himself within a reasonable time.

Regarding minors, the minor is protected by law because he is considered to be under a disability of his minority. The law permits the minor's claim to be extended from the time he reaches the age of majority plus the time specified in the statute of limitations for the particular cause of action. If for example, in a particular state, the age of majority is eighteen and the statute of limitations for a tort action is three years, then the minor would have until he was twenty-one years of age to sue.

Discovery Rule   There is another exception to the statute of limitations and that is the rule of discovery. There are situations where it is impossible for an individual to know he has a cause of action, for example, where a sponge or instrument is left in a patient, or where there is fraudulent concealment of the injury by a health care practitioner. In these and similar types of situations, the statute does not begin to run until the patient knew or should have known of the injury.

Types of Damages

Nominal Damages In a tort injury, an individual seeks redress through monetary compensation for the loss, detriment or damage to the individual's person, property, or rights. There are certain kinds of damages awarded. *Nominal damages* are token compensation where the plaintiff has proven his case but the actual injury or loss is not possible to prove. The customary token award is one dollar. This sometimes occurs when an individual sues for a principle he believes in rather than a desire to be compensated monetarily. For example, a patient who was a Jehovah's Witness sued the physician and the hospital for giving him blood against his will and without his consent. The patient chose to sue based on his first amendment right of freedom of religion and his right to refuse treatment. The patient could have sued on other grounds and asked for compensatory or money damages. Here he only wanted to prove his point—that he had a right according to his religious views to refuse a blood transfusion. The court awarded one dollar as token compensation. Nominal damages are generally not sought in medical-legal cases. The damages usually sought are compensatory damages.

Compensatory Damages *Compensatory damages* are also called *actual damages.* These amounts for proven loss include two areas, general damages and special damages. The *general damage*s include pain and suffering, loss of limb. The monetary value does not always need to be specifically proven. The *special damages* must be proven and include medical expenses, lost wages, sick pay, travel to and from the doctor's office, etc. The law also allows punitive or exemplary damages where the defendant has acted with wanton, reckless, disregard and caused the plaintiff's injury.

If the plaintiff proves his case, the jury will return a verdict in favor of the plaintiff. The jury must then address the issue of damages. The plaintiff presents arguments for the damages he has suffered based on actual damages. In cases where there is temporary or permanent damages, actuarial tables or experts may be utilized to project future losses as a result of injury and these losses are also includable as damages. The jury then decides the dollar amount of the award. Unless the dollar amount is unreasonably excessive, the judge will not interfere in the jury's decision.

CONTRACTS

Definition of a Contract

Everyday we initiate actions that have significant consequences without making a formal agreement. We enter into contractual arrangements in our daily living situations without ever consciously reflecting on the obligations created for ourselves or others. There are certain inferences, expectations and assumptions that everyone makes as part of our daily living. If we were to take the time to reflect, analyze, and formalize such daily living activities, our productivity would be substantially inhibited and ineffective. *Contract* is defined by Black's Law Dictionary as a promissory agreement between two or more persons that creates, modifies or destroys a legal relation. It is also defined as a legally enforceable promise between two or more persons to do or not to do something. In deciding whether a contract has existed, courts have sometimes concluded that a contract was created by a body movement or, in certain circumstances, by the party's remaining silent.

Health care professionals can create obligations which are legally binding under certain circumstances, even though no formal document has been signed. An oral contract is legally binding even though not committed to writing and not formally stamped with a seal.*

Before we can consider the effect and relationship of contract law in our professional life, we must understand certain basic concepts underlying the legal interpretation of what constitutes a valid contract. The first step is to give a legal definition of a contract, then analyze that definition, and proceed subsequently or sequentially from there. To summarize, a contract is a legally enforceable agreement between two or more competent individuals involving a material promise or promises, or sufficient consideration to do or to refrain from doing a particular legal act.

---

* There are certain exceptions governed by the Statute of Frauds which specifically state that certain agreements must be formalized to be legally enforceable. The Statute of Frauds adopted by British Parliament in 1677 was passed to prevent frauds. In essence, it prohibits legal action unless certain contracts are in writing; for example, contract for the sale of land, debts of a deceased, and certain other situations.

Elements of a Contract

The contract is composed of certain parts referred to at law as *elements*. These elements are essential to establishing that a valid contract exists. In analyzing the definition of a contract, the essential elements are: 1) mutual assent, 2) promises or consideration, 3) two or more parties of competent legal capacity, and 4) the agreement must be a lawful act and cannot be against public policy. (See Exhibit 2.)

```
+-----------------------------------------------------------+
|              ELEMENTS OF A CONTRACT                        |
|   Offeror—makes an offer that is    definite               |
|                                     certain        =  A    |
|                                     communicated           |
|   Offeree--makes an acceptance that is  firm               |
|                                         definite           |
|                                         unequivocal  =  B  |
|                                         communicated       |
|                       A + B = C    Contract is created.    |
+-----------------------------------------------------------+
```

Exhibit 2.

Mutual assent means there is a clear understanding between the assenting parties. The law calls it a "meeting of the minds." The offeror, one who makes the offer, and the offeree, one who accepts the offer, must be contemplating the same thing in the offer. The offer is an expression of contractual intent. Therefore, it must be specific, definite, and certain in the terms used to communicate the offer. The power to accept the offer by the offeree can only be created when the offer is definite. Otherwise, there could be no "meeting of the minds." For example, if I offer to sell you my wristwatch for ten dollars, I may be referring to an inexpensive watch that I have at home. But if you think I am referring to an expensive electronic watch I am wearing that appears to be worth considerably more then ten dollars and you say yes to the offer, this is no binding contract. There has not been a meeting of the minds. Therefore, an essential element needed for the construction of a contract is missing. The contract equals offer plus acceptance. However, just as there are certain conditions to be met to establish contractual intent, there are conditions to be met to establish acceptance. The offeree's acceptance must be firm, definite, unequivocal and must meet the specific conditions of the offer when communicated to the offeror. The objective expressed intention of the offeror and the offeree determine if a contract is created.

Consideration is that which underlies and induces the promise or the action. It is the *quid pro quo*, meaning "something for something," referred to at law.

Mentally competent persons refers to parties who are in full possession of their faculties and are not under any legal disability or handicap. Persons who by reason of insanity or who are under the influence of drugs or alcohol or who have not reached the age of majority are incompetent to make a contract. This is an important aspect to be considered in health care situations when patients are asked to agree to procedures or medications or treatments. The possibility that a patient might not comprehend the total situation because of a particular disability must be kept in mind. The particular area of informed consent is dealt with in a separate chapter in this text.

Obviously the law will not uphold an agreement to do an unlawful act. This would be a contradiction in terms. Nor would the courts sanction anything that is against public policy. Therefore, an agreement to do an act that is prohibited by law would not be enforceable. For example, an agreement to procure drugs for a patient in violation of the narcotics law could never be enforced, nor could an agreement to sell stolen hospital equipment. A nurse cannot agree to do what is clearly a medical act since this would be practicing medicine without a license, an illegal act.

The issue, of course, is what constitutes a medical act. Years ago, taking blood pressure or giving an injection was considered a medical act. Today these are acts clearly in the province of nurses, paraprofessionals, and even laymen. But in cases where a particular act is considered to be the province of the doctor, anyone without a license to practice medicine would be prohibited from performing that particular act.

Breach of Contract and Remedies

Because the courts recognize legally enforceable contracts, it gives certain legal remedies for the breaching of a contract. A *breach of contract* is the unjustified failure to perform the terms of a contract as agreed upon or when performance is due. There are generally three distinct remedies for breaching contracts recognized by the law and enforced by the courts. The first is money damages. Take a case where a manufacturer agrees to sell 5000 bottles of a particular medication, such as digoxin, for $500 and the hospital agrees to purchase digoxin according to the terms of the contract. If the manufacturer breaches the contract causing the purchasing agent at the particular hospital to buy the necessary drug at an increased price of $1000, the damages to the hospital as a result of the manufacturer's breach would be $500. Because the hospital had a right to expect to have the contract fulfilled, the hospital has an action at law against the drug manufacturer for the damages of $500 resulting from the breach of contract.

A second remedy for breach of contract is specific performance. This is a situation where the promise or act agreed upon is a special or unique type of performance. Money damages would not be satisfactory. Therefore, the remedy would be to petition the equity court to force or order the party to the contract to specifically perform the promise or act as originally agreed upon. This remedy is usually sought in land contracts or the sale of antiques. Although doctors have the right to refuse to establish a physician-patient relationship with any patient initially, once the relationship is established it is more difficult to terminate. It is conceivable that a doctor who had agreed to perform open heart surgery on a patient and who is uniquely qualified to perform such surgery and who would breach the agreement to do such surgery on a patient could be sued for specific performance. However, the patient would be assuming a risky operation based on many accounts, both the seriousness of the operation and a reluctant surgeon. Nevertheless, the issue would be the remedy of specific performance and the court's ability to enforce the contract assuming all the elements for a valid contract were met.

A third remedy for a breach of contract would be an *injunction*. This is a court order to stop a party to the contract from performing the specific promise or act under other circumstances. The classical illustration is an opera singer who breaches her contract by refusing to perform as agreed upon. The party to the singer's contract on whom the breach was perpetrated could go into court seeking an injunction against the opera singer. The injunction would prohibit her from singing in any other opera house. It is conceivable that where health professionals have agreed at their initial job interview to work at a particular hospital for a minimum of one year and then breach the contract by leaving before the year minimum, an injunction could be sought to prohibit their working in another hospital. As a matter of practicality, administrators of hospitals have not sought a remedy in such situations. However, health care personnel should be aware

Equity court: administer justice according to sense of fairness

that they are bound by the rules and remedies of contractual law and the obligations incurred could be enforced at law.

Oral Contracts   There often is a general misunderstanding that contracts must be written to be valid. As previously stated in this chapter, an oral contract is as binding as a written document (with the exception of the Statute of Frauds as mentioned). However, an oral contract is very hard to prove so; it is good business and better policy to have things in writing. Most attorneys would rather have written documents to present their side of the case than several witnesses who could contradict each other. Even though the witnesses' contradictions might be insignificant, it might affect their credibility with a jury. But, an oral contract that meets all the elements constitutes a binding and enforceable agreement at law. Another misunderstanding is that if a written contract and oral promises were made that are not part of the written contract, these oral promises can be enforced. Oral promises made at the time a contract was signed cannot be legally enforced. Therefore, it should be insisted that all oral terms be incorporated as part of the contract or as an addendum clause.

Classifications of Contracts

Contracts are generally classified as expressed or implied, oral or written. *Expressed contracts* are those where the terms have been agreed upon between the offeror and offeree orally or in writing. *Implied contracts* give rise to contractual obligations by some action or inaction without any verbalization of terms. For example, you have prepared an injection for a patient, you enter the patient's room and say, "Mr. Jones, I have your injection for you." Mr. Jones puts out his arm and you give him the injection. This is an implied consent on the part of the patient. *Oral contracts* are those that are verbally entered into by two or more parties with all the elements of a contract being met. *Written contracts* are those where the elements of a contract are met and the terms of the contract have been reduced to writing. It should be evident that a written contract is preferable to an oral contract, although both may be legally binding.

Contracts and Patients

Health service agencies contract with patients to provide health care services to the patient and the patient agrees to pay a fee for those services either directly or through a third party, such as insurance. This is a *quid pro quo*—something-for-something—arrangement. And if all contractual elements are met, a contract is implied. Because of the nature of health care services in the contractual relationship between the health care agency and the patient, the complexities and variables involved are somewhat different than the average contract for material services. Nevertheless, the health care agency by the very act of accepting the individual as a patient obligates itself to give the standard of care that all other health care agencies in the area give patients. It obligates itself to give due care to the patient and to have competent employees to give that care. The employees who work for the health care agency, although not directly parties to the contract, are indirectly involved in the contractual obligations of the employer.

The patient assumes certain obligations by his admission to the hospital or health care agency. The patient is making a contract when he purchases professional services from the hospital, health care agency, or the health care practitioner. The patient agrees to pay for the professional services and is responsible for the payment even though a third party, such as Blue Cross or Blue Shield, may actually make the payments. The patient agrees to conform to the rules and regulations of the agency relating to patients. It is implicitly understood that the patient will cooperate with the care given by the staff of the health care agency. The patient has the right to refuse any particular care or treatment from any particular person. However, the patient cannot act in a negative manner and disregard hospital policy and then claim damages if injured by his own lack of cooperation. As stated earlier, there is an implied contract each time a patient receives an injection of medication from the nurse. The patient agrees to maintain immobility for the injection and the nurse agrees to give the injection in a competent and skilled manner so as not to injure the patient. This agreement is a quid pro quo interaction. There is no formal written agreement; nevertheless, the patient has assumed the implied obligations of similar patients in similar circumstances.

Liability for patient injury seldom is based on contractual obligations. Liability for patient injury is generally based on the failure of the health care agency or its staff to meet the standard of care due to the particular patient. It is important, however, for health care practitioners to realize that patients have responsibilities and obligations for their health care also.

Contracts with Employers

The employment contract begins with the understanding between employer and employee at the time of the initial interview prior to actual job performance. When the health care professional accepts a job at a particular institution, he has entered into a contract. There is the basic understanding that the health care professional will perform his job competently, safely, and in accordance with the standards and policies of the institution. Also, there is an understanding that the institution will pay for those services, will provide the needed equipment to perform those services, and will maintain the facilities and equipment in a proper manner to encourage efficiency and competency in job performance. There is a mutual obligation on the part of both employer and employee arising from the work contract. Many institutions do not have written contracts. Instead, they choose a general understanding at the time of employment and prefer to have the policy statements serve as a basis for contractual obligations. Although this could be considered poor business practice on the part of both the employer and employee, the courts could still construe a contract from the circumstances under which both parties were working. It is much easier to interpret a written contract of employment than it is to interpret the oral understanding of two parties which may have taken place five or ten years previously.

Often the issue arises where a nurse alleges she was hired with the clear understanding that she would work only in a certain area, such as pediatrics, or that she would have every other weekend off. Subsequently, new rules and policies are established or a new administration comes into the institution. Under the new situation, the nurse is told that she must rotate to a medical-surgical area, or that she will have only one weekend off a month. Before the nurse could be successful in establishing a breach of contract between the employer and the employee she must show that there was a mutual understanding of the particular facts as above, as well as all the other elements of a contract. There must be proof of the existence of such a contract. How easy it would be for the nurse to insist that the conditions of the contract be met if she has a statement in writing to the effect that she was hired to work in pediatrics with every other weekend off. How difficult it is to prove anything where the parties have only their memories with conflicting interpretations of what took place at the initial interview. This does not mean that the law will not enforce a verbal contract. The emphasis is on the difficulty of proving what actually took place.

When the employee claims she was hired to do a specific job and have certain weekends off but lacks written documentation, she does not necessarily lose the case. The courts will generally apply the standard of reasonableness to the situation. In conjunction with the evidence presented by both parties, where certain points are vague or indefinite or controverted, the courts determine what could reasonably be expected to occur and generally construe the contract in that light without any substantive evidence to the contrary.

The question sometimes arises from Directors of Nursing or Directors of Personnel if they are responsible for checking the applicant's credentials, including licensure, graduation, and relevant job qualifications. For example, what if after hiring this individual it was discovered he had a drug problem or that the individual had stolen someone else's license and was not even a licensed professional as purported? It is unfortunate that this and similar situations do occur. However, the legal obligation of Directors of Nursing, Personnel Directors, and those in similar positions is to make reasonable inquiries regarding the credentials of the individual applicant. The law does not place a burden of doing a full investigation on every applicant for a position. Under ordinary circumstances, there is a right to presume that the applicant's credentials are bona fide. Unless there are circumstances which would lead a reasonably prudent person to suspect that the applicant may be a fraud or may be incompetent, you have a right to assume you are dealing with a credible individual. Most health care institutions, like most businesses, have a protocol to follow for reviewing credentials and getting references. If the procedure is followed and is a comparable procedure to similar health care institutions, then the expectations of the law would generally have been met.

It should be noted that a health care institution is a service to the public. Most institutions today are receiving some type of government funding. In today's restricted economy few institutions can function on the fees generated by patient care alone. Where tax dollars are involved in funding or reimbursement of hospital cost, some legal experts consider hospitals to be quasi–public utilities. Therefore, neither the health care practitioner nor the institution can discriminate in the care of the patient. If there are any reservations regarding job performance, they should be made known. For example, a nurse who as matter of conscience does not wish to participate in abortion procedures has a constitutional right to refuse. But she must make this known to administration at the appropriate time, such as the initial interview. If the hospital administration agrees that the nurse does not have to participate in such procedures, then they are bound by that agreement. It becomes a condition of employment and the administration cannot expect the nurse to later participate in abortions. Conversely, the nurse cannot wait until a situation arises and refuse to participate in an abortion. If the refusal or other action would be or could be harmful to the patient, there could be liability incurred for abandoning the patient.

It is good business practice to have the various terms of the contract, such as hours, days off, salary, vacation time and any unusual arrangements, as definite as possible. Whenever possible, make the commitment in writing with a memorandum of understanding attached if necessary. Otherwise, the court may have to interpret any ambiguities.

(See vignettes 17 and 20 for examples of contract situations to validate your understanding of chapter material.)

Case on Contracts

In May of 1974 six students filed suit in the Supreme Court of the state of New York [1] to require the Queensborough Community College Department of Nursing to promote them, alleging breach of contract by the faculty of Queensborough Community College.

The nursing department had decided to upgrade its standards. This particular action was determined to be needed for several reasons. One reason was because of an increased number of students who failed to graduate or did not qualify for advanced nursing courses. Also, there was a definite correlation between students receiving a grade of D or F and those who failed the state licensing examinations.

The faculty of the nursing department were concerned about the quality of nursing care being practiced, so they established a committee to review the issue of grading and quality of care. The faculty committee recommended that a grade of C be required for a student to be promoted in nursing. The faculty council of the college voted to have C as the passing grade in nursing courses.

The students were notified of the change in grading policy. Official notice of the grading change was stated in the 1973/74 college catalogue. Six students who received D grades challenged the legality of the policy and appealed through the appropriate administrative college channels.

The appellate court stated that no breach of contract was involved. A change in grading policy was not a curriculum change. The court construed the catalogue as an informational or advisory document. The court refused to construe the catalogue as a contract between the student and the college. The court ruled in favor of the nursing faculty stating the faculty had a professional responsibility to maintain and improve standards.

1 *Nursing Educator,* September-October, 1976, pp. 22-24.

Labor Relations—Why Do Persons Organize, or Join a Union?

The general reason given for joining a group is to increase power and to be certain of a response from management. Other reasons include clear job inequities that continue unabated unless the employee can assert leverage against the employer to correct the job inequities, such as the need to standardize criteria for advancement, increments, promotion, and benefits. Often the employee is treated arbitrarily or cavalierly by management and has no recourse. Poor communication between the employeer and employee is probably the most basic reason for joining a union. The above reasons, when analyzed, reduce themselves to this basic communication factor. The worker's need for job security, pension plans, and health care coverage also motivates the employee to look for allies in moving management to grant these benefits. It is only in recent years that the health care industry has recognized its obligation to establish pension plans for its employees. Many a health care worker has retired after years of labor only to find he could not subsist on savings and social security. In certain non-profit hospitals even social security deductions were not required for certain employees. This meant those workers were often without any income other than the savings accrued on substandard incomes. Is it any surprise that health care employees could see unions as a type of economic messiah?

Collective Bargaining Under the National Labor Relations Act and Amendments (Effective August 25, 1974)

The 1974 amendment to the Taft-Hartley Act established a procedure for elections and collective bargaining covering nonprofit and voluntary hospitals. This means that all health care workers from aides and technicians to physicians and hospital administrators have a right to be represented by a union in determining certain employment conditions. Through union representation and collective bargaining the individual employee has a stronger voice and more leverage in seeking responses from the employer. By establishing a procedure for collective bargaining, Congress laid a foundation for orderly and civilized resolution of disputes in the health care arena. It is recognized that health care workers, especially those engaged in menial tasks, have long been exploited. They worked long hours at substandard wages. Hospital costs have been increasing for a variety of reasons. One of the reasons not recognized is that health care workers were subsidizing the health care of the nation. Often such workers were expected to substitute dedication for inadequate pay.

There are those who wring their hands and beat their breast crying, "There will be nothing but strikes and increased costs." The fact is that strikes are the exception. No one wants a strike. It is economically injurious for both sides of the negotiations. It is held in abeyance as a last resort. No one wants to suffer economic deprivation. That is what a strike means to both sides of the negotiating table. Employees will lose wages for the term of the strike, be forced to use their savings and very often, even if they "win" the strike, the increase in wages does not make up the lost income. Employers also are not productive during the term of the strike. Consequently profits are decreased. Whether employers win or lose the strike issues, there is always an economic loss.

Employee Representation The National Labor Relations Act provides that whomever the majority of employees in an appropriate bargaining unit designate to represent them, the same shall be the exclusive representatives for collective bargaining. A unit of employees is a group of two or more who share common employment interests and conditions. The determination of an *appropriate bargaining unit* is left to the discretion of the National Labor Relations Board. Generally the appropriateness is determined on the basis of common employment interests. For example, employees with substantially similar interests concerning wages, hours, and working conditions are grouped together. Other factors to be considered by the board in determining appropriateness are: 1) history of collective barganing, 2) desire of the employees concerned, and 3) extent to which the employees are organized.

Bargaining Units The National Labor Relations Board established groupings of hospital employees in the following units:

1. unit of professional employees;
2. separate unit for registered nurses;
3. separate unit for office and clerical employees;
4. separate unit of technical employees to include licensed practical nurses, x-ray technicians, and lab technicians;
5. unit of service and maintenance employees.

The classifications are easily established. What is difficult is the analysis of workers' credentials and functions to fit into those classifications.

The analysis is made according to the criteria of education, skills, and community of interest. The underlying concern of the National Labor Relations Board was to prevent proliferation of units. The organizing of many units makes the entire mechanism of collective bargaining unwieldy since there would be continuous negotiations with numerous splinter groups.

The *majority exclusive representative principle* is that the representative or union selected by a majority of employees in an appropriate unit for bargaining would be the exclusive bargaining representative for that unit of employees in the hospital. Otherwise every individual group with a vested interest would want recognition. This would mean that hospitals and health care facilities would be engaged in collective bargaining with one group or another continuously and would not have time to perform their primary function —quality patient care.

These groupings have caused much controversy and concern. Health care workers who have considered themselves professionals see the groupings of the Board as a derogatory commentary on their competencies. Licensed practical nurses, in particular, view their separation from the registered nurses' unit as a weakening factor for both organizations. What the ultimate effect on all health care workers will be remains to be assessed as litigation of cases occurs.

Units and Supervision   The term *supervisor* has been used very broadly in the health care field. One employee demonstrating a procedure to another has been termed to be "supervising a procedure." Another employee placed in charge of a health care unit for a limited time has been termed a supervisor. Charge nurses, floor unit managers, and even team leaders have been referred to as "supervising employees" in health care institutions. This broad construction of the term supervisor is not compatible with the more narrow definition given by the National Labor Relations Board. A *supervisor* as defined by the statute is one who hires, fires, transfers, suspends, lays off, recalls, promotes, discharges, rewards, or disciplines employees, or is responsible for directing employees, or adjusting grievances or actively recommending any of these actions.

This definition of the word "supervisor" is crucial to nurses. When it is realized that the interpretation means that certain nurses would be granted or denied union membership based on the construction of the term, the significance of the definition is more fully appreciated. Under the act, supervisors are not "employees." As a result "supervisors" cannot be included in employee labor organization units for negotiations or collective bargaining purposes. Another significant point is that the supervisor is considered to be an agent of the employer. The supervisor acts for, on behalf of, and in place of the employer. It is as though the employer were doing the particular acts and the acts of the supervisor are imputed to the employer. Therefore, any activity engaged in by a supervisor that could be construed as an unfair labor practice would be imputed to the employer (hospital or health care institution). The old adage, "no one can serve two masters" is clear. It would mean an obvious conflict of interest which could not be permitted.

The determination of who is a supervisor is still somewhat ambiguous in the health care setting. The board has given a definition which serves as a guideline. However, in the health care setting, application of the definition depends on the facts and circumstances of each particular case. There is more complexity of tasks and overlapping of functions and responsibilities in health institutions than in industrial areas.

Significant Differences for Health Care Facilities   In passing the 1974 amendment, Congress had special concerns when giving collective bargaining rights to nonprofit hospitals. Congress was concerned that there be no untoward effect on patient care as a result of the new legislation. Congress advised in its legislation that a reasonable accommodation be made regarding strikes. Employees in health care institutions may strike after following all appropriate procedures and giving the employer a ten-day notice of intention to strike. This is done to allow the employer adequate time to make contingent plans to care for patients in order that essential or critical care needs will be met.

Another difference is the *ally doctrine* as it relates to health care areas. In order to understand the ally doctrine, we must address ourselves briefly to the *secondary boycott* concept. They are closely related but distinct concepts. A secondary boycott occurs if a union has a dispute with Med–Instrument Supply Company who makes dressings, syringes, and hospital equipment. To strengthen their dispute, the union causes employees of Community General Hospital to stop handling products manufactured by Med-Instrument Supply Company or otherwise force Community General Hospital to stop doing business with Med–Instrument Supply Company. The dispute is with Med–Instrument Supply Company who is called the "primary" employer. The union is taking action against Community General Hospital who would be considered the "secondary" employer and there-

Imputed: **ascribed vicariously to person**

fore the term secondary boycott. The Labor Relations Act forbids secondary boycott as unfair labor practice on part of the employee. Such unfair labor practices can result in a union losing its recognition as the exclusive bargaining agent.

The ally doctrine is differentiated from the secondary boycott in the following manner. Let us say that Med–Instrument Supply Co. who makes dressings, syringes, and hospital equipment is engaged in a strike. Med–Instrument Supply Co. makes an agreement with Sleak Surgical Supply Co. who makes dressings, syringes, and hospital equipment to supply Community General Hospital for the term of the strike. Sleak Surgical Supply would then become Med–Instrument Supply Co.'s ally in the union dispute and would be subject to union action also. This would be acceptable and legal union activity, in ordinary industrial labor relations. In the health care field we are not dealing simply with commercial commodities. Primarily, health care facilities are dealing with essential and critical health care needs and human lives. Congress has recognized this fact. Therefore, if one health care institution is struck, it is acceptable and legal to request assistance from other health care institutions. These other institutions do in fact become allies under the act. But because of the type of care and assistance given, that is, critical help or facilities, the institutions giving such help are protected from being picketed or struck by congressional mandate. A caveat to the health care institutions, the key term is *critical* or *essential* assistance. The protection does not extend to noncritical assistance such as clerical or ward clerk or other similar activities. Attempts of assistance of a non-essential nature could be construed as inappropriate and illegal and result in union action against the ally institutions.

It is interesting and commendable to note that Congress recognizes the complexity of health care institutions and has given special considerations to their problems in enacting labor relations legislation in health care areas.

Grievance Procedures   In the American tradition of fair play, grievance procedures are becoming an essential part of every organization's policy. It has always been a part of our judicial system that an individual is innocent until proven guilty. It is also part of our system that everyone is entitled to his day in court. The grievance procedure merges these two themes as part of the process to give employees justice and equity in their employment. Any employee who believes he has

Caveat: warning

been treated unfairly or arbitrarily can seek justice or redress through a grievance procedure. The grievance procedure is a tribunal set up on an informal basis to hear employees' problems and reach a decision regarding those problems. It has the essence of the American judicial system without all the formalities. Generally, the employee presents his grievance before a hearing officer. The employee often represents himself and presents his own case. Where a union is recognized or certified by the organization, the union representative presents the employee's case. The administration or management is generally represented by a member of management or an attorney or both. Each side presents witnesses or evidence to support their contentions and to rebut their opponents' case. After hearing both sides of the dispute, the hearing officer gives his decision and recommendations. This decision can either be accepted or appealed. If either side decides to appeal the decision of the hearing officer, they may continue to the next step of the process. Generally, the final step is binding arbitration which means the decision made by the arbitrator must be accepted as final on both sides.

As always, there is still a right to go to court. If a particular appellant has followed the grievance procedure appropriately and has exhausted all his administrative remedies, then he may go to court. Generally, the courts are reluctant to overturn or reverse a decision made by the proper persons in a grievance procedure. The appellant must show that the decision of the arbitrator was arbitrary and capricious and not simply that the decision was not to the appellant's liking.

Discipline Discipline and behavioral correction should be a continuous process in any organization. It should not be sporadic or related to favoritism or other irrelevant criteria. Employers are justified in disciplining employees who break rules or ignore policy. One of the criticisms of unions is that you cannot get rid of incompetent employees where unions are present. This is not a valid statement. The issue is quite often lack of documentation. You may not be able to get rid of an incompetent employee on the basis of the naked allegation alone. What you must do is substantiate your statements. There must be factual proof and evidence of the employee's incompetence. If there is sufficient proof, then generally the union will not prevail. It may take longer to build a case against an incompetent employee

Appellant: party who takes appeal
Arbitrator: one who decides disputed issues

but it can be done. The union can prevent arbitrary and capricious dismissal of employees. The union cannot prevent that dismissal where the facts and evidence are clearly presented in an objective and non-prejudical manner. Where the employee has been given a proper hearing and due process of law, and the facts are such that reasonable men would conclude the employee is incompetent, the union would be dilatory in supporting the employee.

Part Two
CONTEMPORARY LEGAL-MEDICAL ISSUES

EVOLUTION OF THE RIGHT TO HEALTH CARE

The health care professions have a humanistic tradition. The Code of Hammurabi, 2000 B.C., was the earliest set of regulations to govern the health professions. The nursing and medical professions, like every profession, are guided by a code of ethics. This code of ethics is mandatory for every practicing member. The code is basically a recognition of the rights of individuals and the respect due to these individuals undergoing health care. It also incorporates the ethical guidelines to which these professionals are expected to conform while acting as a health care practitioner.

The complexity of health care has contributed to the complexity of ethical-legal decisions. Social values are irrevocably interrelated with health care and with the ethical-legal decisions involved in that health care.

There are certain rights protected by society and by law. The term *right* by definition means a claim to which an individual is entitled. The right is recognized by a court of law and enforceable. The decisions of the courts reflect the values of society at large. Recently, judicial decisions have been significantly dominated by social issues and public policy.

There has been a dominant movement in the area of patient's rights in the health care field. For every legal right there is a corresponding duty to recognize the right and not to interfere with the individual's exercise of the right.

The main thrust of arguments for patient rights is based on the fact that every individual is entitled to certain basic rights as a human being. Patients do not waive any of their rights simply because they become patients. There have been great strides in this area to assure that patients entering health care facilities are not denied their basic human rights. The majority of these rights are based on constitutional, statutory, common law, or contractual rights. Health care practitioners must recognize and respect all the patient's rights and not interfere with the free exercise of those rights.

Courts and Health Care Rights

The courts have been accused of effecting social change through judicial mandate. Constitutional lawyers who are strict constructionists of the United States Constitution claim that the courts have acted beyond their constitutional authority in making decisions that have the effect of making law which is a legislative function, rather than interpreting law which is a judicial function. Other legal experts argue the courts are interpreting law in the light of contemporary issues and setting precedent, that precedent being that quality health care is a constitutional right.

Regardless of which legal expert is correct, there is no doubt that judicial decisions have made an impact on enforcing individual rights granted by the United States Constitution and state legislatures. There have been achievements of equal rights for minorities and now the time has come to give equal justice and protection to a minority that is not often recognized as a minority—the patient. This patient group is split into even more unfortunate minorities of the elderly, the abused, the handicapped, and the dying.

The term *handicapped* is broader than the traditional interpretation of mentally retarded. To be handicapped is to be disabled, to be placed at a disability. Anyone who is a patient, whether in an institution or at home, is essentially handicapped. If you or a member of your family had experience as a patient, you will accept the premise that a patient is handicapped in many ways when moving through the health care system.

Health Care Delivery System and Patient's Rights

Health care delivery systems often intimidate the patient. It is ironic that professions which profess to be humanitarian and concerned with dignity of the patient have had to be censured for running roughshod over basic rights of individuals, alias "patients." Health practitioners who would be indignant that a citizen's free speech or right to vote would be endangered in a democratic society do not hesitate to ignore a patient's right to make his own medical decisions. Every day in health institutions, we find patients disenfranchised of their voting right, not because they have committed a felony but because they are admitted or committed to a health agency. It is basic to the care of all patients in any environment that all persons dealing with patients understand that no patient or health care consumer waives any rights, constitutional or otherwise, when he enters a health care system.

All persons, minorities and handicapped, are entitled to first amendment rights—freedom of religion, thought, expression, and communication.

All persons, minorities and handicapped, are entitled to the fifth amendment rights—due process of law.

All persons, minorities and handicapped, are entitled to the sixth amendment rights—to have access to an attorney, to face their accusers and to have a proper judicial hearing.

All persons, minorities and handicapped, are entitled to the eighth amendment rights—to be free of cruel punishment from personnel caring for them, or in treatment, which includes the right to refuse experimental treatment or behavior modification treatment or chemotherapy. What of the mental and physical deterioration which often follows commitment to mental institutions?

Finally, all persons, minorities and handicapped, are entitled to the 14th amendment rights—equal protection for all citizens.

If you do believe that all citizens have these rights under the United States Constitution, then it is self-evident that your approach to all consumers of health care will reflect this belief. And logically, you will be an advocate of the patient's right to quality health care and self-determination in matters of personal health care.

Contemporary Issues

The following section deals with patient's rights in general and specific contemporary issues in which patient's rights are considered in relation to the public right or interest.

The federal government project which was begun over forty years ago in Tuskegee, Alabama, has emphasized the need to protect patients. This was a study on 399 victims of syphilis who were all black and who were told they were participating in a health program. Most of the patients had less than a sixth grade education. The true purpose of the study was to determine the long-term effects of syphilis on persons who had received no treatment for it. None of the participants in the study were told the true purpose of the study.

In New York City in the late 1960's, elderly patients were injected with cancer cells without their consent, indeed without their knowledge that they were being subjected to such research. In the early 1970's in New York, a group of mentally retarded children were given injections of fecal extract containing a hepatitis virus. Again, consent was not solicited and these children were victims of assault and battery among other things. There are other examples, not antiquated ones but situations that have occurred in this twentieth century, and not in Nazi Germany but in our own democratic America.

What can be said of a system that permits such abuse and violation of a human person? Where are the built-in monitors to prevent such exploitation and experimentation of "handicapped" persons? Is the "educationally handicapped" patient being violated in the name of scientific progress? But those examples are the extreme inhumanities. What of the simple health care rights to which a patient should be entitled? The patient should have a right to know the medication he is receiving and the interactions of other food and drugs on his system as a result of the medication. The patient should have access to his medical records in the best interest of his health and well being. In short, the patient should have complete and final jurisdiction over his health care unless there is a conflict with the social or public interest. Yet, patients are often relegated to the role of passive observer in their own health care and sometimes not even consulted before treatments or procedures are done on and to them. These kinds of actions cannot be countenanced by any health care practitioner. A nurse is a patient's advocate *de facto* if not *de jure*. It is up to the nurse to protect the patient's rights if the patient is unable or incapable of protecting those rights himself.

Self Evident Rights and Rights in General

It is a somewhat sad commentary on the health profession that a patient bill of rights must be committed to a statement in writing

De facto: in fact, actually, reality, thus an office, position or status existing under a claim or color or right
De jure: by act of law

or to legislative enactments. These rights should be self-evident. The simple fact is that patients are entitled to dignity, consideration, and self-determination.

Many state legislatures have passed a patient's bill of rights document either as a resolution or as statutory law. Some jurisdictions have limited the patient's bill of rights to nursing homes and others have extended it to all health care facilities. Minnesota has enacted legislation which requires the patient's bill of rights be posted in all hospitals. The Minnesota statute states that anyone who intentionally abuses or culpably neglects a patient is subject to a fine of $1,000 and up to a year in prison. This type of statute with a punishment clause elevates the patient's bill of rights to more than a strong statement of philosophy.

It has been necessary to develop a commitment to patient's rights, to reiterate to the staff and the public that patients are human beings with the right to be treated with dignity and consideration. The health agency is in existence to serve the patient. The patient did not come into being to serve as a hospital commodity, teaching, or research material for the health care system.

The rhetoric surrounding the care of a patient generally is aimed at creating a public image of great concern for the health care consumer. The philosophy, bylaws, policies, and newsletters of the institutions are filled with statements of the institution's goal in achieving quality care. There are several diverse elements converging on the patient as he seeks treatment in the maze of preventive and therapeutic medicine. Because of the present complexity of the system and some of the abuses which have been disclosed, it is necessary to inform the patient of his rights while undergoing care. The patient should be made aware that he has the right to accept or reject treatments recommended to him, the right to privacy, the right to be free from unnecessary risk of injury, and the right to be the prime determiner of what is to be done with and to his body. A *right* has been defined as a claim to which a man is entitled. A right is, by its nature, recognized by law and enforceable in a court of law. It would follow that the patient's bill of rights can only have credibility if recognized as capable of being enforced in a court of law and as a subject of legal redress for patients.

These factors, plus the nurse's and physician's pledge to give quality health care and to establish an environment in which the patient can exercise all his constitutional rights, are significant factors

Culpably: deserving blame

in ethical-legal issues. There are important legal and ethical issues to be resolved as the implementation of the patient's bill of rights takes place.

There is a consensus that the purpose of the patient's bill of rights was to reaffirm the concern of health care practitioners for the patient's human dignity. This reaffirmation is a new commitment to quality health care for all citizens and marks a new revolution for all health care consumers. The Constitution of the United States is a viable document and must be operative in all health care facilities for all patients.

Some additional specific contemporary ethical-legal issues presented in this section that deal with patient's rights are abortion, the right to die, child abuse, involuntary commitment, informed consent, confidentiality, and invasion of privacy. There are other issues, but these topics have been selected as the most important and controversial.

The following is an example of a patient's bill of rights, published by the American Hospital Association:*

1. The patient has the right to considerate and respectful care.
2. The patient has the right to obtain from his physician complete current information concerning his diagnosis, treatment, and prognosis in terms the patient can be reasonably expected to understand. When it is not medically advisable to give such information to the patient, the information should be made available to an appropriate person in his behalf. He has the right to know by name, the physician responsible for coordinating his care.
3. The patient has the right to receive from his physician information necessary to give informed consent prior to the start of any procedure and/or treatment. Except in emergencies, such information for informed consent, should include but not necessarily be limited to the specific procedure and/or treatment, the medically significant risks involved, and the probable duration of incapacitation. Where medically significant alternatives for care or treatment exist, or when the patient requests information concerning medical alternatives, the patient has the right to such information. The patient also has the right to know the name of the person responsible for the procedures and/or treatment.
4. The patient has the right to refuse treatment to the extent

* Reprinted with the permission of the American Hospital Association.

permitted by law, and to be informed of the medical consequences of his action.

5. The patient has the right to every consideration of his privacy concerning his own medical care program. Case discussion, consultation, examination, and treatment are confidential and should be conducted discreetly. Those not directly involved in his care must have the permission of the patient to be present.

6. The patient has the right to expect that all communications and records pertaining to his care should be treated as confidential.

7. The patient has the right to expect that within its capacity a hospital must make reasonable response to the request of a patient for services. The hospital must provide evaluation, service, and/or referral as indicated by the urgency of the case. When medically permissible a patient may be transferred to another facility only after he has received complete information and explanation concerning the needs for and alternatives to such a transfer. The institution to which the patient is to be transferred must first have accepted the patient for transfer.

8. The patient has the right to obtain information as to any relationship of his hospital to other health care and educational institutions insofar as his care is concerned. The patient has the right to obtain information as to the existence of any professional relationships among individuals, by name, who are treating him.

9. The patient has the right to be advised if the hospital proposes to engage in or perform human experimentation affecting his care or treatment. The patient has the right to refuse to participate in such research projects.

10. The patient has the right to expect reasonable continuity of care. He has the right to know in advance what appointment times and physicians are available and where. The patient has the right to expect that the hospital will provide a mechanism whereby he is informed by his physician or a delegate of the physician of the patient's continuing health care requirements following discharge.

11. The patient has the right to examine and receive an explanation of his bill regardless of source of payment.

12. The patient has the right to know what hospital rules and regulations apply to his conduct as a patient.

ABORTION

Whatever one's reaction to the term *abortion,* it is seldom neutral. Begin to discuss abortion and normally rational persons become quite emotional and react strongly. Abortion is defined by Black's Law Dictionary as "the expulsion of the fetus at a period of utero-gestation so early it has not acquired the power of sustaining an independent life." Webster's Dictionary defines abortion as "the expulsion of the mammalian fetus prematurely, before it is viable." Taber's Medical Dictionary defines abortion as "the termination of pregnancy before the term of viability, that is, before the 28th week." As common law, any individual who intentionally committed an act to end a pregnancy prematurely, that is, before the age of viability, was guilty of a crime. If the pregnant woman died during the attempted abortion, the perpetrator of the abortion could be charged with the crime of murder or manslaughter depending on the intention or knowledge of the perpetrator performing the abortion. There has been a long legal and ecclesiastical prohibition on birth control, sterilization, and abortion. But societal pressures and recent court decisions have removed many of those prohibitions. There are strong voices and arguments being heard both for and against abortions. Although the Supreme Court has ruled that a woman has a fundamental right to an abortion in the first trimester of pregnancy, the "Right to Life" advocates are moving to counter this decision with constitutional amendments to protect the rights of the fetus in utero.

There is controversy and debate over the subject of abortion because it is not an isolated subject. The medical, legal, ethical, social, economic and cultural elements of society are inextricably woven into the issue of abortion. Everyone is affected, either directly or indirectly, in some way by the positions taken on this controversial subject.

Arguments Related to Abortion

The arguments advocating abortion are persuasive. There is the illegitimate child who may be subjected to cruelties and harassment from peers. There is the young mother who may be subjected to emotional trauma and possibly overwhelming infections from an illegal abortion. The young mother herself may be hardly more than a child

Perpetrator: person who commits a crime, or by whose agency the act
occurs

attempting to raise a child. There is the family who simply has too many children to adequately provide for them. There is the growing welfare caseload of unwanted children who are economic burdens on taxpayers. There is the tremendous guilt complex to which women are subjected as a result of society's attitudes toward sexual promiscuity. Advocates of abortion argue that women will have abortions regardless of the consequences. It is better to provide proper facilities, qualified personnel, and help the individual rather than to criminalize her. In recent years, environmentalists have warned that if voluntary contraception and abortion are not encouraged, coercive measures may become necessary to control population. The key argument favoring abortion states simply a woman should have the right to determine for herself what happens to her body.

The adversaries of abortion point out that it is purely and simply an unjustified homicide. Their argument is that science has identified "life" and therefore the potential for a meaningful existence outside the uterus early in the first trimester. If life occurs at the moment of conception, then the potential person is entitled to all constitutional rights. The anti-abortionists argue that the fetus is the most vulnerable and unprotected of all minority groups. They also argue that abortion on demand is the beginning of the end of a civilized society.

Decisions on Abortion

The present law of the land as promulgated in the landmark Supreme Court decisions of *Doe v. Bolton* [1] and *Roe v. Wade* [2] is that every pregnant woman has a constitutional right to have an abortion during the first trimester (12 weeks) of her pregnancy. *Griswold v. Connecticut,* [3] 381 U.S. 479 (1965) was a landmark case involving the use of contraceptives. The Griswold decision held that a state statute making the use of contraceptives a criminal offense was unconstitutional. It stated a woman had a fundamental right to bear a child or not bear a child. Such a statute was an unconstitutional invasion of the right of privacy as it relates to sex and marriage. The Supreme Court based its decision on the fourteenth amendment concept of liberty and right to privacy.

The Court [4] in the case of *Roe v. Wade* held that state statutes which prohibited abortion were unconstitutional. This case originated

1 *Doe v. Bolton,* 410 U.S. 179, (1973).
2 *Roe v. Wade,* 410 U.S. 113 (1973).
3 *Griswold v. Connecticut,* 381 U.S. 479 (1965).
4 *Roe v. Wade.*

in Texas. The Supreme Court through the Roe decision held that during the first trimester, the pregnant woman has a constitutional right to an abortion and the state has no vested interest at that time. During the second trimester, the state may regulate abortions. These regulations should be reasonable and related to the health of the pregnant woman. During the third trimester and especially the final 8 to 10 weeks of pregnancy the state may regulate and proscribe abortion to protect the rights of the fetus. But if continuation of the pregnancy threatens the health or life of the mother, an abortion is indicated and the state must allow it. The main issues in the Roe case were whether the right to personal privacy includes the right to have an abortion and whether the fetus is a person, according to the constitution, entitled to all constitutional rights. The court concluded that the right to an abortion was absolute in the first trimester and became qualified or limited as the viability of the fetus developed. The court ambiguously stated that viability might occur as early as the twenty-fourth week, but usually occurs by the twenty-eighth week. The Roe court, speaking through Justice Blackmun, stated that the fourteenth amendment protection of the constitution does not apply to the unborn. The consideration of the ethics and legality of fetal research is raised by the court's ruling. If the fetus is not a person protected by the 14th amendment, then it could legitimately be subjected to investigation and research. Would it or should it be considered as property belonging to the bearer of the property, and necessitating consent of the bearer or appropriate monetary compensation for use of the property? Or is it simply disgarded waste similar to other waste products of the body and therefore fair game for experimentation and not even subject to the Nuremburg code.[5] There are strong pro–life group movements throughout the country who advocate constitutional amendments to restrict or prohibit abortion. The basis for their arguments is that life occurs at the time of conception and the embryo or fetus is then a person entitled to constitutional protection. They point to the progressive and cumulative scientific evidence that the fetus has human characteristics and functions at early development.

The Supreme Court decision addressed the issue of spousal consent. The court held that the consent of the married father to an

Proscribe: prohibit

[5]   The Nuremburg code evolved as a result of the Nuremburg trials in post World War II Germany. It prescribed certain criteria to follow during research and human experimentation.

abortion is not necessary and any requirement of such consent is unconstitutional. The courts in general are moving in the direction of not distinguishing between minor pregnant women and adult pregnant women.[6] Based on social and health policy, an absolute parental consent requirement would probably result in minor pregnant women seeking other alternatives such as criminal or self-induced abortions. The Supreme Court has stated that parental rights are not absolute but must be balanced against the rights of the child and the interests of the state.

What is the health practitioner's responsibility with regard to abortions? Very simply, the health practitioner is obliged to follow the law. It has now been established by the Supreme Court that a woman may have an abortion as a matter of right under the 14th amendment as previously stated. Each state may vary the time restrictions in the second and third trimesters as previously indicated. It is now the law of the land and no one is above the law. If any health practitioner does not wish to participate in performing abortions or preparing patients for abortions because of religious, moral or personal reasons, he has no legal obligation to do so. There is generally a "conscience clause" in this type of legislation. This means that any person who would be acting against their individual conscience of right or wrong by participating may conscientiously object and no redress or liability would result.

It has been the authors' experience when discussing this topic with health practitioners that the health practitioners had difficulty separating their conscience from the patient's conscience. A health practitioner has no right to use his religious or moral views as a guide in caring for a patient. When it is pointed out to the health practitioner that a nurse would not hesitate to care for a drug addict or a patient with venereal disease without passing a moral judgment or attempting to infer that they not be given treatment, this sometimes aids the health practitioner in getting his functions back in proper perspective.

The authors do not for a moment intend to suggest that a health practitioner should condone abortions if this goes completely against the ethics which the practitioner follows in daily practice. But the authors do suggest that a health practitioner legally has no right to condemn the patient by word, act, or attitude because the patient elects to have an abortion. This is quite difficult for health practitioners, especially those who work in the delivery rooms or obstetrical out patient departments of hospitals. They argue that in one room of the

6   *Coe v. Gerstein*, 376 F. Supp 695 (S.D. Fla. 1974)

delivery suite, doctors and nurses work to save the life of a newborn, while in another room of the same suite, a suction machine is being used to complete an abortion. There is no question that this is an absolute paradox, yet the role of the health practitioner is clear. He may choose whatever course his conscience dictates, but he cannot impose his conscience onto others.

CHILD ABUSE

Definition of Child Abuse

Child abuse can be broadly defined as the malicious beating, striking, or otherwise mistreating of a minor under the age of 16 years to such a degree as to require medical treatment for such a child. The term child abuse is a generic term covering broad areas of mistreatment.

There is considerable variation in the statutory language throughout the United States. More than twenty of the states, including the District of Columbia, refer to physical injuries inflicted by other than accidental means. There are some states that consider intention, or willfulness, an essential element for child abuse to be a crime. Some states clearly differentiate between neglect of a child and abuse of a child. Other states use broad language and indicate that any injury to a child resulting from some act or from some omission where there is a duty to act regardless of the willfulness or intent will be considered criminal.

History

Historically, the state has been reluctant to interfere with the family unit. This is not peculiar to the parent-child relationship only; it was also true of the husband-wife relationship. The courts, until recently, viewed both wife and child as "chattels" or property of the husband or father.

The mistreatment of children and infanticide have been a part of history since before the hieroglyphics of Egypt. Infanticide was an ancient ritual to bring rain, sun, good harvests, health, wealth, and all material pleasures. Children have been subjected to varied treatment in the name of religion, progress, and societal needs. It was commonplace in certain cultures to sell daughters into prostitution and sons into slavery. With the advent of the industrial revolution, large families could prove to be a lucrative enterprise as children were pushed into the factory system at early ages. Compulsory school attendance was unheard of during the advent of industry and children were forced to spend long hours at hard manual labor in the "sweat shops." The prevalence of child abuse historically makes total elimination of such treatment unrealistic. But certainly alleviation and consciousness of the problem is not beyond achieving in this century.

Beginning Legislation

The abuse of children is not a recent sociological phenomena. The "battered child syndrome" is a new term used to describe an ancient situation, the misuse and unconscionable beating of helpless children. History is full of incidents of children being sold by parents similar to selling any piece of property. Children have been sent to work at jobs unfit for adult employment in factories, on farms, and other hard labor areas. There were no child labor laws to protect the child and 10- or 20-hour work days were not unusual terms of employment for a young, unloved child. Aside from the child labor laws to protect the working child, there was little legislation. The first laws calling for mandatory reporting of child abuse resulted from a 1963 Children's Bureau Report.[1] Most states had protective legislation by the early 1970's but there was no standardization and much diversification. The first model legislation for the states on child abuse and neglect was published by the Early Childhood Project Education Commission in 1973.[2] The Child Abuse and Treatment Act[3] was also enacted in 1973. The act resulted from Senate hearings on child abuse. The act required that states meet certain uniform standards to be eligible for federal assistance in setting up programs to identify, prevent, and treat child abuse problems. It also established a national center on child abuse and neglect.

The act stipulates that state statutes must require mandatory reporting of abuse and neglect and mandatory assignment of a *guardian ad litem* in all abuse cases.[4]

The abuse of a child is considered to be a criminal act in most states and therefore involves criminal sanctions of either fines or im-

---

1 Children's Bureau, U.S. Dept. of Health, Education and Welfare, *The Abused Child—Principles and Suggested Language for Legislation on Reporting of the Physically Abused Child* (1963).
2 Early Childhood Project Education Commission, *Child Abuse and Neglect: Model Legislation for the States* (1973).
3 *Child Abuse Prevention and Treatment Act,* Act of January 31, 1974, Published L. No. 93-247; 88 Stat 4 (1973).
4 Public Law No. 93-247, Section 4(b) (2) (B).

prisonment or both. Other states place child abuse in a non-criminal category, not necessarily because the state considers the act of child abuse less serious but because the state does not believe the criminal process serves a useful or beneficial purpose for the child or parents involved. For example, the stigma or fine resulting from a criminal conviction often does irreparable harm to the family and a fine further reduces an often low income. It is believed the public and other appropriate persons would report violations of child abuse more often and quicker if criminal sanctions were not involved.

Distinction Between Abuse and Neglect

The superficial distinction between abuse and neglect is that *abuse* generally is an affirmative action on the part of the parent or adult and *neglect* is the failure to act. Also, abuse is usually of a greater degree. While courts generally differentiate between abuse and neglect, as a practical matter and for remedial or punitive treatment, the psychopathology of neglect and abuse appears to be significantly different in assessing the potential for rehabilitation.

The phenomenon of abusing and mistreating children, minors or *non compos mentis* persons is a historical fact not confined to twentieth century America. There are numerous historical references to the widespread pervasiveness of mistreatment of the more vulnerable elements of society. During the 18th and 19th centuries, children were considered to be the property of the father. They could be mistreated or used at the father's discretion as any other property he owned and the child had no protection. This was the era Charles Dickens immortalized in the classic *Oliver Twist* and which a recent broadway show, "Oliver," portrayed.

It is difficult for the average citizen to understand the extent of the child abuse in our society. It is hard to conceive that an adult or parents could deliberately and knowingly abuse a helpless child. Child abuse has existed in all societies for centuries. In spite of this, even today, communities and health professionals are not aware of the children who are victims everyday of emotionally disturbed parents who take their frustrations out on their own children. As the statistics are

Ad litem: for the purposes of the suit
Guardian ad litem: a guardian appointed to prosecute or defend a suit on behalf of a party incapacitated by infancy or otherwise

compiled on a nationwide basis, the full horror of child abuse is placed before the medical and legal disciplines to seek solutions. Sixty-thousand cases of abuse were reported to the National Center for Prevention of Child Abuse in Denver, Colorado.[5]

Profile of a Child Abuser

Studies thus far indicate that the parent or adult who abuses once will be repetitively abusive. The classic picture is that of an individual who intends to correct or teach a child. The correction is extended and the adult or parent loses control and ends up maltreating the child.

The developmental pattern of the adult or parent who is abusive is one of frustration, hostility, suppressed aggression, and poor self image. The irony is the abusive adult is often the product of abusive parents also. More and more studies indicate that abusive parents are emotionally immature, tragic personalities themselves. After there is assurance that the children in the situation are protected, attention should be directed to the needs of the abusing adult. Research data compiled by Dr. C. Henry Kempe [6] of the National Center for Prevention of Child Abuse and Neglect in Denver, Colorado, shows that every strata of society produces "battering parent" types. It is not limited to low income groups. The data demonstrated that the battering parent distrusts authority figures, had one or more aggressive parents, had a poor self-image, needs constant reassurance, and tends to become violent when this reassurance is not received. Dr. Kempe believes that a majority of abusive parents can be rehabilitated with therapy. The center followed a mothers anonymous program similar to alcoholics anonymous. It is a type of crisis or emergency center where a parent can go for help if he or she feels overwhelmed in trying to cope with his child or children. Help is available around the clock. This center holds that with proper treatment and a coordinated supportive program for the parent, children can be returned with no repeated abuse or violence.

In contrast to this concept of rehabilitation, Peter De Courcy, a clinical psychologist, sees little hope for the abusive parent. In his book, *A Silent Tragedy*, he documents multiple instances of brutal treatment of children. From his study, De Courcy states that child

[5] A National Symposium on Child Abuse, presented in Rochester, New York, October 19, 1971.

[6] Friedman, S. B., "The Need for Intensive Follow-up of Abused Children," *Helping the Battered Child and His Family*, C. Henry Kempe and Ray E. Helfer, Lippincott Co., Philadelphia, Pa., 1972.

abusers have severe personality disorders making them poor risks for rehabilitation.

The term "battered child syndrome" was coined during the early sixties. Although the medical profession had been aware of unexplained injuries occurring to children, medical personnel were reluctant to characterize the condition and notify proper authorities to prevent further abuse or harm coming to the child.

The reality of child abuse, child neglect, and sexual exploitation of children has only begun to receive public attention in recent years.

In many cases, the suspected abuse of children is not sufficient reason for removal of the child from the home. But it frequently warrants protective supervision for the child. This supervision is generally a specialized service given by the social welfare agency in a state. Counseling with the parents and coordinating services for parents and children are the core of most programs. The main objective is to develop behavioral changes and appropriate attitudes in the parents.

Reporting Suspected Child Abuse   Two common denominators throughout child abuse legislation are that a social welfare or law enforcement bureau should serve as the resource for reporting of abusive incidents and that any parties reporting incidents of abuse or suspected abuse would be immune from being sued. The latter, obviously, is a critical factor because health professionals in some instances were reluctant to report suspicious cases because of fear of being sued in the event the charge was proven untrue. The immunity provision is necessary to protect these persons whose only purpose is to protect the child and who are making a *bona fide* report. It is not intended to protect those persons who would harass parents.

The fear of being sued for slander or malicious prosecution resulting from initiating charges against a parent was a major reason given by doctors, nurses and concerned citizens for remaining silent about possible child abuse. However, because of the increasing number of cases in this area and the reluctance to assist law enforcement agencies in prosecuting "abusive parents," the majority of states have passed legislation known as the *child abuse statute*. These statutes give immunity from suit to persons who report suspected child abuse to appropriate authorities based on evidence or facts that would cause a reasonable person to suspect a child had been physically mistreated or abused. (An example of a child abuse statute is found in the appendix.) All of the states have some type of legislation which requires child

Bona fide: in good faith

abuse to be reported. But passage of a law does not guarantee its implementation nor the solving of the problem for which legislation was passed. Before enactment of child abuse statutes with an immunity clause for those reporting these abuses, medical persons and private citizens were reluctant to make the moral commitment necessary to see a child abuse case through to a conclusion.

Now the sad commentary is the lack of awareness on the part of health care practitioners that a child abuse law exists. How can such a law designed to be protective of the child be effective under such circumstances? There are some states that enumerate those persons required to report suspected child abuse and grant immunity from liability if reported in good faith. There are other states, such as Arizona, Florida, New Jersey, New York and Pennsylvania, which impose a penalty on certain categories of persons for not reporting suspected child abuse. The Federal Standards *require* mandatory reporting of child abuse cases.

An interesting case, decided upon by the California courts, could conceivably result in criminal or civil liability for failure to report suspected child abuse. In a 1976 medical malpractice case in California,[7] a child, Gita Landeros, was repeatedly beaten by the mother and the paramour. The child had been taken to a local hospital on at least two occasions. Gita had several fractures, bruises and contusions over parts of the body and the mother gave no creditable explanation for the child's condition. No report was made to the appropriate legal authorities, and the child was sent home with the mother. Approximately a month later, the child was hospitalized again with more injuries. The child was diagnosed as a "battered child" and legal proceedings were initiated. Gita Landeros, through her attorney, sued the emergency room physician and the hospital for failure to diagnose and report the condition of the battered child to the appropriate legal authorities. It was the contention of Gita's legal representative that their failure to act responsibly and appropriately resulted in her being subjected to further injury. This injury could have been prevented by timely reporting to legal authorities. The Supreme Court of California ruled that the emergency room physician and the hospital may be held liable for injuries received as a result of the failure to diagnose and report the child abuse to local officials or proper legal authorities.

The other prong of the legislation includes systematically gathering statistical data on child abuse incidents by having a central registry system. Most states have moved in this direction. The registry serves other purposes such as detecting repeated offenders.

---

[7]   *Landeros v. Flood,* 131 Cal. Rptr. 69, 551 P. 2d 389 (1976).

Public Education

Health care practitioners should be educating the public about child abuse. The legislative intent of the Child Abuse Prevention and Treatment Act (public law no. 93-247) was to encourage health care institutions to develop innovative programs to identify, report, and most important, prevent child abuse. Consumer-patient education programs could be developed to teach the symptoms, diagnosis, and treatment of child abuse comparable to the health teaching of diabetics or cardiacs in hospitals today. Continuing and in-service education programs for staffs should be promoted in this important area so the public as well as professional staffs are clearly aware of their role and responsibility in relation to child abuse prevention.

Some Indications of Child Abuse

The heterogeneousness of abusive parents ranges from the illiterate to highly educated; from laborers to professionals; from the poor socio-economic level to the affluent. All races, religious, and ethnic groups have the dubious distinction of being represented.

The strongest evidence that shows one is dealing with the classical "battered child syndrome" are x-ray findings of repeated bone injuries. X-rays which reveal bones healing at different stages indicate that injuries occurred at various times. It is logical to assume this type of multiple injury results from deliberate abuse and not by accident. This is not necessarily sufficient evidence to find a parent guilty "beyond a reasonable doubt" in criminal court. But it is sufficient evidence to have the protective juvenile services investigate and evaluate the family unit.

As to sexual abuse, the majority of sexual offenders of children are members of the child's everyday environment—a relative, a neighbor, a friend of the family. In a New York study, the sexual offender was frequently the father of the female children. And even more pathetic, the researchers were convinced the mothers were fully aware of the situation in many instances. There are many cases which go completely undetected because of the age of the victim and the setting in which the act takes place. Because of our criminal procedures, the emotional impact on the sexually abused child is often compounded when detected rather than alleviated. A child must testify in detail under oath in open court to the sordid event.

Some legal experts question the advisability of continuing child abuse as a criminal act. The theory is that if it were a civil offense, the public is more likely to respond and report, therefore affording a higher degree of protection to the child. The child abuser could still be subject to criminal prosecution and subject to other criminal laws such as assault and battery. Also, the child would not be subjected to criminal procedures to establish proof of the incident. The test would be by a preponderance of evidence as required in civil actions, and not beyond a reasonable doubt and with a moral certainty as required in criminal law.

Conclusion

There is no greater need for preventive medicine, instead of therapeutic aid, than there is in the field of abuse of children. All personnel handling pediatric emergencies should develop an awareness that traumatic injuries, such as burns, dislocations, fractures, head injuries, abrasions, bruises, and nosebleeds, are to be considered as high risk types of injury often found in victims of child abuse. Therefore, they should be primed to pick up any significant data relevant to this often overlooked clinical entity.

A young battered child who comes to the clinic or emergency room is extremely fortunate to be treated by an intern or nurse or para-professional who is alert enough to analyze the situation. It is difficult for anyone to be absolutely certain that he is facing a case of child abuse. Legislatures, therefore, have couched the language by saying "has reason to suspect" what a reasonable person would infer from the evidence before him. The language of the law is quite broad. Its desire to protect the child even at the risk of wrongly inferring the guilt of the parent clearly exists.

Professional persons in the health field who have the responsibility of caring for children are required by law to report suspected child abuse to the proper authorities. They have an obligation as skilled health care professionals to detect incidents of abuse or repeated abuse. Lack of knowledge of symptoms of child abuse or reluctance to become involved are no excuses for not fulfilling one's obligation under the law. The health practitioner may be the only advocate the abused child will ever have.

Case on Child Abuse

United States of America v. Martha L. Woods,
U.S. Court of Appeals, 4th Circuit, September 1973

This is a case involving the ultimate in child abuse. Martha L. Woods was found guilty of first degree murder of her eight-month-old foster son, Paul David Woods. Paul was born February 9, 1969, and spent his first five months in a foster home without any physical problems. Paul was placed with Martha Woods in July, 1969. Beginning August 4, 1969, a bizarre series of events occurred. On August 4, 8, 13, 20 Paul suffered episodes of dyspnea and cyanosis. He became comatose on August 20 which persisted to September 21, 1969, when he died at seven months of age.

During the trial, the government presented evidence that, beginning in 1945, Mrs. Woods had custody of nine children who suffered a minimum of twenty episodes of cyanosis. Seven children died, while five had multiple episodes of cyanosis.

There was a sanity hearing prior to trial. It was concluded that she was capable of being tested. There appeared to be no motive for the alleged murder. The burden of proof was on the government to prove beyond a reasonable doubt that Paul's death was caused by culpable homicide perpetrated by the defendant. They introduced a brief history of the nine children mentioned above with emphasis on their health and illness histories.

The courts permitted evidence of the events in the lives of the other children to be admitted to demonstrate a pattern of circumstantial evidence. The court held that when the crime is one of infanticide or child abuse, evidence of repeated incidents is especially relevant because it may be the only evidence to prove the crime. A young child is a helpless, defenseless unit of human life, too young to relate the facts concerning the attempt on his life. The court reviewed evidence of abuse in each of the nine children's cases. It concluded that if the evidence regarding each child is considered separately, some incidents are less conclusive than others; but when the incidents are considered collectively, an unmistakable pattern overwhelmingly establishes the defendant's guilt. The defendant was sentenced to a total of seventy-five years.

The main issue in this case was obviously that of proof. It is always difficult to sustain a case of child abuse because there is seldom an eye witness to such abuse other than the victim. But it is necessary to be aware that persons can be convicted of crimes that they have not committed as well as never be charged for crimes they have committed.

When the case was appealed, Judge Widener dissented from the majority opinion. Judge Widener was convinced the defendant did not receive a fair trial. He said that admitting evidence of prior occurrences was inflammatory and prejudicial. He further stated that testimony offered by the government of prior incidents involving children other than Paul D. Woods was improperly admitted. Judge Widener reviewed the same evidence presented to convict the defendant and concluded there was not sufficient evidence for a conviction. In fact, it was the evidence that was left out; where were the autopsy reports on the other children who had died?

This case serves to illustrate the difficulties involved in prosecuting a child abuse case diligently and appropriately, but above all, with all the fairness of judicial process.

DIGNIFIED DEATH

There is concern and confusion over the individual's "right to die." Members of the legal and medical professions are both antagonists and protagonists on the various issues related to the subject. It raises more controversy than the emotionally charged issue of abortion. One thing is certain, everyone is going to die and will therefore be affected by decisions relating to dying. Everyone is not going to have an abortion so the vested interest in that subject is lessened. The *thanatology* era is in full bloom in the United States today. Thanatus is a Greek word meaning death. Courses on college campuses, television documentaries and newspaper series explore the subject and give rise to a death consciousness in society today. There are sociological and economic implications in prolonging or shortening life that have caused unprecedented philosophical controversy.

Euthanasia is a Greek word translated as "an easy and painless death." Euthanasia does not mean "mercy killing" as is often misunderstood. Because of the frequent misunderstanding and misinterpretation, the Euthanasia Society of America changed its name to the Society for the Right to Die.[1] This appears to be more acceptable terminology.

Early history establishes that suicide was permitted. St. Augustine has been identified as one of the first to teach that suicide was both a sin and a crime. In England for many years, anyone attempting or committing suicide was punished by having his property and land seized by the state. After a substantial time, Parliament realized it was the family that was being punished by such procedures and not the perpetrator of the suicide. Parliament then repealed the law. There are still cultures today that both condone and encourage the

[1] Joel Goldberg H., "The Extraordinary Confusion Over 'the Right to Die,'" *Medical Economics,* Jan. 10, 1977, P. 122.

taking of one's life under certain circumstances. For example, in World War II, the kamikaze [2] pilots were trained to perform suicidal missions by crashing into the designated targets. This was considered an honorable feat. If the kamikaze pilots failed in their mission, they would commit suicide because they were dishonored and disgraced.

Traditionally, the American system of jurisprudence recognizes the sanctity of human life. The taking of the life of an innocent human being is absolutely forbidden. Moralists, ethicists, and jurists have recognized the justifiable taking of life in certain circumstances. Life may be taken during war, in self-defense, and where society decrees it as punishment for a crime. These and similar circumstances would be considered justifiable homicide. The premeditated killing of a human being without justification is murder. *Murder* is the taking of a human life accompanied by the element of deliberateness, malice aforethought, and premeditation. *Manslaughter* is the unlawful taking of a human life without malice. It is done while committing an unlawful act. It is done unintentionally or in the heat of passion where capacity to form intent is diminished. Manslaughter is classified as voluntary and involuntary. *Involuntary manslaughter* is the unintentional taking of human life while committing an unlawful act. *Voluntary manslaughter* is the taking of human life in the heat of passion when suddenly provoked.

There are moral, ethical, and legal issues related to death by choice or death with dignity that would puzzle King Solomon himself. Paul Ramsey, a professor of religion at Princeton University, believes there is a moral obligation "to care for the dying and never to hasten the dying beyond the reach of our love and care." [3] But Professor Ramsey admits that there are exceptions where the patient is entirely indifferent to the method by which his dying is accomplished. The implication in the exception seems to be that where there is irreversible mental damage and the patient is unable to formulate a concern for the method of his dying, some acceleration of the process should be

Jurisprudence: philosophy of law or science which treats the principle of positive law and legal relation

[2] Kamikaze—The pilot of an explosives laden Japanese plane whose sole mission was a suicidal crash dive upon a target, especially a ship.
[3] Paul Ramsey, *The Patient as Person* (New Haven and London: Yale University Press, 1970), P. 162.

permitted. Richard McCormick, an ethicist, declares that "taking life is wrong, unless there is a proportionate reason to do so." [4] The exception to the prohibition of accelerating death by a positive act is again admitted to by a prominent ethicist. But what is a "proportionate reason to do so?" Who is to establish the standards and criteria of a "proportionate reason" to satisfy the value judgments of society at large?

Sanctity of Life

Conventionally and traditionally our health care system has been permeated with the *sanctity of life* principle. This hippocratic oath sworn to by physicians implies the affiant will do everything to benefit the sick and to preserve life. This approach to death and dying is being re-examined. There are many philosophers, physicians, lawyers, patients, and laymen who believe the time has come to replace the concept of sanctity of life. The main arguments presented by such revisionists are that it is not always the kind and loving thing to do to preserve life. In fact, they argue that there are times when love and kindness demand the taking of a human life. *Ethics* has been defined as the science relating to moral action or moral value. *Moral* has been defined as normatively human, what is expected of humans, that which humans ought to do.[5] *Law*, according to Black's Law Dictionary, is that which must be obeyed and followed by citizens, subject to sanctions or legal consequences. In the triumvirate of moral, ethical, or legal considerations, the law would subject the lawbreaker to punishment. Therefore, it is prudent for any health practitioner to consider the effect of the law on any selected actions surrounding death with dignity situations. The challenge to health care practitioners, legal experts, and society as a whole is to develop moral, ethical, and legal situations compatible with contemporary needs. This expectation may be unrealistic, but it is the only intelligent approach to the controversial health care issues of present day society.

Affiant: one who swears to a statement

4 Richard McCormick, *Ambiguity in Moral Choice,* the 1973 Pere Marquette Theology lecture, Milwaukee: Marquette University Theology Publication, 1973, P. 95.
5 Daniel Maguire, *Death By Choice* (Doubleday and Company, Inc., Garden City, New York, 1974), P. 77.

What Is Death?

Death is the termination of life. The problem arises in ascertaining the termination of life. How is that determination to be made? In ancient times, death was probably crudely established by the lack of breathing and body movement for a period of time. In the early 1900's, the cessation of breathing and the lack of a heart beat and pulse beat would bring a pronouncement of death. Today a newer criterion has been introduced, that of brain death. Dr. Julius Korein of New York University School of Medicine includes in his definition of death the "destruction of that critical component of the system which represents the essence of the person and which cannot be replaced with . . . auxiliary support systems." [6]

Some authorities argue that there should be some type of mechanism for a definition of death that is precise and allows a patient to be pronounced dead while still maintaining "life" for purposes of organ and tissue transfer. According to some experts, this would create over 10,600 organs for needy recipients.[7] This attitude addresses itself to the humanistic or materialistic need for donors. It does not consider the related moral, ethical, and legal implications.

Father Thomas A. Wassmer, a Jesuit theologian, states that there is no legal definition of death based on present day medical facts.[8] The cases in recent years, notably the Karen Ann Quinlan case to be discussed later in the chapter, brought the realization that the medical issue of death was unattended by legal definitions and that physicians could be placed in the position of committing an illegal act by removing life-supporting systems inappropriately. Today the legislatures of all the states have moved to define and clarify the meaning of death.

Kansas [9] was the first state to enact legislation to determine medical and legal death. In general, the statutes equate human life with the function of the brain. In the absence of brain function, a person is dead irrespective of the function of other organs. The statute was criticized because it listed alternative definitions of death. A special committee in California addressing itself to this issue concluded the

---

6   "On Cerebral, Brain, Systemic Death," in *Current Concepts of Cerebrovascular Disease: Stroke,* a publication of the American Heart Association, Inc. 8, No. 3 (May-June 1973): 9.

7   Maguire, *Death By Choice,* P. 18.

8   Thomas A. Wassmer, "Between Life and Death: Ethical and Moral Issues Involved in Recent Medical Advances," Villanova Law Review 13 (1968): 776.

9   Kansas Statutes annotated, Sec. 77-202, Supp. 1971.

important issue was "to establish the legality of the concept of death" [10] not necessarily the specificity of it. There continues to be voluminous discussion on the absence of "quality of life" as an abstract criteria for determining death. But most states are moving to the statutory brain death concept accompanied by a protocol to determine that death. The protocol generally consists of a flat electroencephalogram and absence of reflexes and similar criteria.

Uncertainty about the legal definition of death has contributed to the anxieties of physicians, families, and potential patients who are faced or may be faced with life and death decisions. States are moving in the right direction by enacting more definitive statutes pertaining to death.

Death by Choice

The main issue in the right to die with dignity is the moral, ethical, and legal issue of whether an individual has the right to terminate his own personal life or the life of another under certain special circumstances. The first basic premise in assessing dying patients is that every individual reacts to the process of dying in a unique manner. The uniqueness is a result of an individual's frame of reference developed over a lifetime. It is inaccurate to assume that anyone given the choice of living a few months in pain and suffering or having their life terminated by humane medical procedures will opt for death. Studies [11] have shown that dying patients have not been given the opportunity to express themselves. Those same studies also indicate that patients want assistance to go through the dying process and not necessarily to have the process abruptly terminated.

The right to die with dignity rather than be subjected to unnecessary pain and suffering is a right which everyone agrees every citizen should be afforded. How this right is to be implemented or enforced is a matter on which a consensus is improbable. Euthanasia (good death) is classified as voluntary or involuntary, active or passive, direct or indirect. *Voluntary* implies a willful act or intention as opposed to *involuntary* or unintentional. The *active* and *passive* classification refer to taking positive action to terminate life as opposed to doing nothing to assist a patient to prolong life. The *direct*

10   "Statutory Brain Death?" Department of Pathology, University of Southern California, Los Angeles, Journal of the American Medical Association, August 26, 1974. Vol. 229, P. 87.
11   Elisabeth Kubler Ross, *Questions and Answers on Death and Dying*, MacMillan Publishing Co., Inc., New York, 1974, PP. 76-78.

and *indirect* aspect also refer to the procedure or manner of terminating life. Voluntary, active, direct death by choice would be suicide by gunshot or hanging. Involuntary, passive, indirect euthanasia would be removing the respirator and similar life support systems from a patient.

Negative, passive, or indirect euthanasia usually refers to not using any extraordinary means to prolong life. The commission and omission dichotomy is an integral part of the controversy surrounding the right to die issue. The majority appear to accept that not doing anything to prolong life as acceptable and moral. But to act, that is, a commission to end a life by a lethal injection, is met with charges of murder. Yet, on analysis, the decision to end a life and the decision not to do anything to prolong a life have the same intention and the same goal. As early as 1957, Pope Pius XII [12] stated that a respirator is not morally obligatory for a patient in a hopeless state of unconsciousness. The respirator, according to the Pope, could be turned off under these circumstances. The question which the Pope did not address is whether the turning off of a respirator is an active or passive act, an act of omission or commission.

Opponents of euthanasia—the right to die—argue the "domino theory." The domino theory states that if mature adults choose to die rather than select unbearable or unacceptable alternatives, it will be the beginning of the end. The dominoes, representing handicapped, elderly, retarded human beings, will fall one after another until the choice of who shall live or die will be decided on arbitrary physical criteria. Opponents believe the sanctity of life will be devalued when euthanasia becomes acceptable. They are absolutely opposed to death by choice because they believe the foreseeable effect is genocide or mass killing of defective or handicapped human beings. Viable alternatives can only be explored on a case method. Some patients want to die because life has no meaning. An individual given options might choose to live. The key word is *viable*. In other cases induced death may be selected over protracted pain and suffering.

Proponents do not claim there will be no abuse of death by choice, but they argue that every competent adult should have the right to choose death over prolonged pain and suffering. Proponents also argue that all mature adults do have the right to refuse all extraordinary means of life support equipment and that this right should be recognized and respected by health care practitioners.

---

12 "The Prolongation of Life, an Address of Pius XII to an International Congress of Anesthesiologists," November 24, 1957, the Pope speaks, 4, No. 4 (1968), P. 397.

The conscious, competent, terminal adult individual who has the right to refuse medication, to leave a health care institution against medical advice, and to decide the degree to which he will cooperate in his health regime is the same patient who should be able to control the final decision of his life—how to die.

As previously stated, all dying patients do not react in the same way. A patient dying with terminal illness may choose to be kept alive in the hope of a cure or for religious or other reasons. Another patient may choose to discontinue all medications, chemotherapy, treatments or procedures. Another patient might choose to select terminating his life by receiving a lethal injection.

Legislatures have attempted to pass euthanasia statutes as early as 1937 in Nebraska, New York, Connecticut, Idaho, Wisconsin, and Florida, while other states have attempted legislation unsuccessfully. The first "natural death act" (California health and safety code section 7185-7194, 1976) to be passed was in California when Governor Edmund Brown, Jr. signed the Landmark Bill on September 30, 1976. The act, which became effective January 1, 1977, authorizes among other things the withdrawal of life-sustaining procedures from adult patients with a terminal condition where the patient has executed a "living will." Further, the California legislature gives its citizens the right to authorize the physician to withhold life-sustaining procedures which artificially prolong life. The key element in the natural death document is that the section titled "directive to physicians" must be executed under specific conditions. This places certain restrictions and presumably protections in the law. The written authorization becomes operative when and if the individual is certified terminally ill by the attending physician and another independent physician.

The executed directive is effective for five years. The qualified patient must be examined and certified by two physicians for terminal illness and the directive or living will must be witnessed by two objective, unrelated witnesses.

The increased impetus to the right to die bill is the Karen Ann Quinlan case. The case clearly illustrated the issues of ordinary and extraordinary means, legal definitions of death, quality of life and prolongation of life by artificial means. These and other similar questions had never been considered in the state of New Jersey. As the nation followed the progression of the case, it became clear that few, if any, states would be prepared to answer similar situations.

Karen Ann Quinlan was placed on a respirator after being admitted in an unconscious condition to a hospital in Morristown, New Jersey. It became evident that the respirator was merely keeping Karen alive. Neurosurgeons and other specialists agreed Karen was only vegetating and was incapable of any cognitive functions. Mr. and Mrs. Quinlan made the decision to request the court in New Jersey to order that Karen be removed from the respirator and allowed to die in dignity. People across the nation identified with the issues in the case. Some believed that to take Karen off the respirator would be a positive act, an act of commission and, therefore, homicide. Others believed it would be merely an act of omission, a passive act, and simply cessation of extraordinary means. Judge Muir ruled the law of the state of New Jersey precluded the removal of Karen Ann Quinlan from the respirator. Judge Muir [13] indicated such an authorization would have been in conflict with the statutory law of New Jersey and would be a homicide. He further stated that humanitarian motives would not be sufficient justification for the taking of a life.

Mr. and Mrs. Quinlan appealed the unfavorable verdict of Judge Muir. On March 31, 1976, Judge Hughes [14] speaking for the Supreme Court of New Jersey ruled the termination of treatment, pursuant to the right of privacy, was permitted under the circumstances presented in the Quinlan case. He further stated there was a determinative distinction between the unlawful taking of a life of another and the cessation of artificial life-support systems.

There are several cases where the life of a person suffering from a terminal illness or in great pain has been taken by a family member. Often the victim has asked to be relieved of pain permanently. In case after case, the jury has listened to all the evidence and returned a verdict of "not guilty by reason of insanity." It seems where the defendant is charged with mercy killing, the jury utilizes its prerogatives to acquit the defendant. For the jury to rule an act to relieve a loved one from suffering as murder, a premeditated killing, is a disparity they cannot accept. In 1967, the jury could not equate Robert Waskins with a murder. Robert was the 23-year-old son whose mother was suffering from leukemia, who was in pain and begged him to relieve her of that pain. Robert took his mother's life. The jury acquitted him.

Making the Decision

It is generally conceded that any competent adult should have jurisdiction to answer the famous Shakespearian question "to be or not to be," to live or not to live. But where an individual is in a coma or a state of irreversible unconsciousness with no reasonable

13   *In re Quinlan*, 137 N.J. Supp. 227 (1975).
14   *In re Quinlan*, 355 A.2D 647 (1976).

hope of recovery, who shall make the decisions affecting that individual's right to live or die? Who should decide? By what authority should the decision be made? What criteria should be utilized? What are the implications for the individual affirming or denying another's right to life? The authors do not suggest any answer to these awesome questions. Instead, the authors suggest some considerations about each potential decision maker. The first person usually suggested to decide is the physician or a group of physicians. The doctor has no special competence for such a decision simply by reason of being a medical doctor. The doctor may not be aware of significant personal issues surrounding the patient and the patient's family. The "medical mystique" should not be allowed to prevail and give physicians automatic jurisdiction simply because they are doctors. Their advice on the medical aspects is obviously needed, but the possibility of conflict of interest in making an objective judgment for the patient's best interest would negate consigning such a decision without guidelines and controls.

What of a special advisory committee? Several hospitals have moved in this direction. The committee composition is varied. It is usually an interdisciplinary committee. Currently, such committees have no legal power to authorize the removal of life-supporting equipment. They serve to assist the family and physician to arrive at the decisions they must make.

What of the family deciding? The family should not be too quick to abdicate their role to the presumed higher knowledge and ability of the health care professions and the courts. On the other hand, the family might be emotionally overwhelmed and unable to make such a decision. Perhaps the family might feel forever guilty if electing to remove life-sustaining equipment and have doubts about the decision long after it has been made. Also, one must consider that during lengthy illnesses even the most loving families could wish to be relieved of the economic burden of a protracted dying patient and opt for removal of life-sustaining equipment for vested interests.

What if the patient designated a particular individual to make such a decision in anticipation of such an event or possibility? The law permits persons to act as *agents* and *alter egos* at other times. If a person chooses an individual, tells that individual his wishes, and authorizes the individual to act in his best interest, why should the courts, the health care profession or anyone else interfere? Such a

Agent: person authorized by another to act for him
Alter ego: other self

plan and procedure would save the family from the emotion of this final decision. It would be more objective because there would be no benefit inuring to the decision maker. The individual would have been designated by the patient and therefore presumably acting in the patient's best interest. As with any situation, if anyone believed the decision maker to be acting improperly or illegally, the courts could be called upon immediately to review the decision.

There is great concern over 1) the right to die with dignity being codified and becoming the law of the land with all its implications, and 2) the designating or consigning of the decision to the appropriate decision makers. This chapter raises many questions and gives few answers. The only answer that can be given is one's own answer to the question. Then, paralleling Patrick Henry, we know not what course others shall take but as for us; we want to make all our own decisions just as long as we possibly can and especially the one about dying; we would not give that awesome decision to anyone but one of our own choosing.

THE PATIENT'S RIGHT TO KNOW

Doctrine of Informed Consent

This could more appropriately be called the patient's right to know and participate in his own health care. *Informed consent* is a doctrine that has evolved sociologically with the changing times. The courts have mandated that every patient is entitled to an informed consent before any procedure can be performed. Judge Benjamin Cordozo, while serving on the court of appeals of New York in a 1914 case,[1] stated that every adult has a right to determine what is to be done to his body. He said a surgeon who performs an operation without the patient's consent may be liable for assault and battery. An assault is the threat to do bodily harm to an individual. The act of doing the physical harm is the battery. It is therefore necessary for patients to consent to surgery or medical procedures in order for a charge of assault and battery to be avoided.

Consent   It is basic that the intentional touching of another without his consent could be construed as a legal wrong constituting assault or battery or both. *Consent* is the affirmation by the patient to have his body touched by certain designated individuals such as doctor, nurse,

---

1   *Schloendorf v. Soc. of New York Hosp.*, 211 N.Y. 125, 105 N.E. 92 (1914).

laboratory technician, or others. There are different classifications of consent as discussed in an earlier chapter. There is the implied consent. When a patient rolls up his sleeve to receive an injection, this action can be construed as a consent to the procedure. An expressed consent, as the term implies, is an affirmative action or statement to signify his intention.

There are also the verbal and written consents. An oral or verbal consent is binding. The problem arises when it comes to a question of *evidentiary matter*. It might be difficult to prove the patient gave an oral consent. Even where witnesses are present and hear the consent given, their testimony might not be consistent on details and could weaken their credibility. A written consent obviously offers some tangible proof that the patient voluntarily signed a form. It is subject to scrutiny and disbelief if other facts relevant to the situation indicate that the patient did not fully and intelligently understand what the affixing of his signature meant in relation to his medical care.

A proper consent form is an important evidentiary document in the event of a dispute regarding the claim that an informed consent was not given. The signed consent would generally be considered presumptive evidence that an informed consent to a particular act was given. It is a rebuttable presumption. But the burden of proving the consent was not given would be upon the patient.

The individual giving consent must be mentally competent and able to appreciate the material facts. The patient must have consented freely and voluntarily, based on sufficient knowledge and information to make an intelligent decision.

The necessary elements to constitute valid written consent must include the patient's signature attesting that the procedure to be performed was the one to which he consented and evidence that the person consenting understood the nature of the procedure, the risks involved, and the probable consequences. The explanation of the procedure should be in understandable terms. Technical and complicated explanations should be avoided.

Rescinding Consent The patient may rescind the consent given either verbally or in writing at any time. A written consent may be rescinded verbally. Any time a patient withdraws his consent, it is as though he had never given a consent. This means that any procedure done on a patient who has rescinded his consent would be a battery.

Evidentiary matter: any species of proof, or probative matter presented by the act of the parties for the purpose of inducing belief in the minds of the court or jury as to their contention

Who May Consent

Normal Procedure   The patient upon whom the procedure is to be performed is the only one who has authority over his body as long as he is conscious and competent. It is essential to respect the individual's right to make his own decisions. Health care practitioners often bypass obtaining consent from an elderly patient whose only impediment is grey hair or telltale signs of aging and ask the son or daughter to give consent. It cannot be overemphasized that an adult who is mentally competent is the final authority over decisions that affect his health care and his life. Hospitals, health agencies, or health care practitioners cannot arbitrarily be substitution decision makers. The next of kin or family members or anyone else cannot consent for a patient who is mentally competent. If the person is mentally incompetent, consent must be obtained from a person legally authorized to give consent for the patient. For example, an elderly or infirm person may have had the foresight to authorize a power of attorney designating a child or relative to act in his behalf. In the case of a person declared legally insane, authorization for medical care should be obtained from the mentally incompetent's committee established by law.

Spouse's Consent   Confusion exists in the area of consent regarding husband and wife. Can a husband consent to his wife's operation in a non-emergency situation? The answer is clearly no. Is the husband's consent also necessary in operations involving reproductive organs where some marital interest might be involved? The answer is still no. And the converse is true. The wife has no authority to consent for the husband. The individual upon whom the operation is to be performed is the sole determiner. No one can give permission to have surgery performed on another. This area has become confused because doctors and hospitals often have the husband and wife sign operative permits as a matter of policy and precaution. It then takes the tenor of law in the hospital, and personnel interpret the policy as though it were statutorily mandated. It is probably good business to have a spouse sign the consent forms. This could then serve as one piece of evidence if a dispute arose later regarding the consent and might prevent needless litigation. But it is not legally mandated.

In a 1974 case [2] a husband sued the physician for performing a

Power of Attorney: an instrument authorizing another to act as one's agent

[2]   *Murray v. Vandevander*, 522 P. 2d 302 (Ikl. App. 1974).

hysterectomy on his wife. The husband alleged the operation interfered with his marital rights and was done without his consent and with notice of his specific disapproval to the surgeon. The Oklahoma court ruled that a married woman is not required to have her husband's consent to receive health care. The court said the right of a competent person to consent to procedures regarding his own body is the transcending right.

Minors Consent A minor is considered to be under the jurisdiction of his parents until he reaches the age of majority. The age of majority is the statutory or legal age of adulthood. In most states that age is eighteen years. In general, the parents or legal guardians of minors are authorized to consent to medical treatment and procedures. There are certain exceptions to this general rule. Most states have enacted legislation which permits minors to consent to certain medical treatment and procedures as though they were adults. The statutes vary slightly from state to state. But in general, the minor may consent for his own care if married, emancipated, pregnant, suffering from a venereal disease, or in need of psychological or psychiatric care. The term *emancipated* means the individual is no longer under the control of another. The emancipation of a minor child means the child no longer seeks the care and custody of the parent. Generally, this occurs where the minor is working and is responsible for his own support and necessities. If this is established, the law generally recognizes the minor as one entitled to be treated as an adult with all the rights of an adult including that of consenting to health care.

Consent to Medical Treatment The common law holds that the natural parents or legal guardians of a child have the authority to consent to medical care for the minor. Historically it has been held that a minor is immature, inexperienced, and incapable of making appropriate decisions. The parent is presumed to act in the best interest of the child, and therefore there is a presumption that the child will be protected. This is a rebuttable presumption. There are times when parents, because of religious belief, will not permit the child to receive medical care that society believes is in the child's best interests. In these circumstances, the state must exercise its right under the *parens patriae* doctrine and intervene to protect the health of the child. The state, on occasion, has intervened by ordering a blood transfusion to preserve the life of the child.

Parens Patriae: duty of state to protect its citizens

Emergency Situations In an emergency situation anyone may do whatever is necessary to preserve life. The law implies that the victim in an emergency would want everything done to save his life and protect him from harm. An emergency generally exists where there is a threat to the life or health of an individual that is sudden and immediate. In such an event, an individual or health care emergency team may do what is believed necessary without an expressed consent on the part of the patient or his family. The consent is implied by law. There would be no liability regarding the consent. It would be appropriate and good policy to keep the next of kin informed and to get their approval if possible, but it is not legally required. In summary, the emergency rule applies where the person is in immediate danger of death or serious bodily harm and is incapable of giving consent.

Informed Consent

Stated briefly and succinctly, an *informed consent* is one in which the patient has received sufficient information from his physician concerning the health care proposed, its incumbent risks, and the acceptable alternatives to that care so the patient can participate and make an intelligent, rational decision about himself. Some recent cases illustrate both the criteria used by the courts in deciding if an informed consent was given and the reaction of the court to the physician meeting or not meeting that criteria. A recent California [3] case places the responsibility of getting that patient's informed consent on the doctor. It is stated as a *fiduciary duty*. Ralph Cobbs underwent a gastrectomy for ulcers and developed complications. Although the patient, Ralph Cobbs, was told the type of operation he was to undergo and the possible risks of the general anesthetic he would receive during the operation, he was not told of the possible risks and complications involved in the surgery itself. Following discharge from the initial surgery, Cobbs was readmitted for emergency surgery of a severed artery. Cobbs sued both for negligence in the performance of the surgery and for failure to obtain an appropriate consent. The jury ruled in favor of Cobbs, awarding a $45,000 verdict against the hospital and a $23,000 verdict against the surgeon.

The hospital and doctor appealed. The Supreme Court of California found there was insufficient evidence to support the jury's conclusion that the physician had been negligent. The court ordered a new trial. In ordering a new trial it set out certain guidelines to be followed by the trial court rehearing the case. The Supreme Court of Califor-

[3]   *Cobbs v. Grant,* 104, 229 Cal. Rptr. 505, 502 P. 2d I (1972).

nia, among other things, said that the physician-patient relationship is a fiduciary relationship. That is, the physician has certain expert knowledge and the patient trusts and relies on this expertise. The physician has a duty of disclosing as much information as the average reasonable person, in the same set of circumstances as the patient, needs to decide if he wants to accept or refuse the proposed surgery or procedure. The physician does not have to go into remote possibilities of serious bodily harm that might occur. But where it is common knowledge that there are inherent risks of death or serious bodily harm, the doctor has a responsibility and an obligation to tell the patient and to explain in layman's terms the complications that might occur. The patient should be able to make an intelligent decision about his body. The court said the patient's right to self-decision is the measure of the information needed and what information is material.

There also has to be a causal connection between the failure to inform and the injury suffered. This is established when it is shown that if the patient had more relevant information about the treatment and its inherent risks, the patient would not have consented to the treatment or procedure. The amount of information necessary to meet these standards varies with the facts and circumstances of each case.

In another consent case, Mrs. Pegram,[4] a 35-year-old mother was experiencing abnormal vaginal bleeding. Her doctor did a cervical conization and a pap smear. The diagnosis was early squamous cell cancer. Her doctor advised her to have a radium implant and referred her to a Dr. Sisco. Mrs. Pegram was admitted to Springdale Memorial Hospital and the operation was performed.

Mrs. Pegram testified that no one before, during, or after the radium implant procedure ever explained anything to her. She also developed a large vaginal-rectal fistula which caused feces to be passed vaginally as a result of the operation. She eventually had a radical hysterectomy and colon resection operation.

Essentially she alleged that neither the private physician nor Dr. Sisco ever explained the basic procedure of the radium implant, nor did anyone inform her of the alternative procedures available, such as a hysterectomy. There was no information given or received regarding the possible complications of radium.

The court ruled from the evidence presented that there was no informed consent obtained in spite of the fact the patient had signed a

Fiduciary: position of trust

4 *Pegram v. Sisco*, 406 F. Supp. 776 (D. Ark. 1976). ,

standard consent form. The court said such a consent is ineffectual unless the person knows the dangers of the procedure to which he consents. Dr. Sisco was found negligent in treating the patient by not following community medical standards which might have prevented the resulting fistula. Dr. Sisco did not make an adequate disclosure of the radium implant procedure, its attendant risks, and effects. He also did not tell Mrs. Pegram what other alternatives were available in order for her to make an intelligent decision.

In the Martin Case,[5] the physician did not apprise the patient fully of the risks he would be subjected to. Mr. Martin received emergency treatment at Lutheran Hospital following severe injuries to his hand resulting from an accident with a butcher knife. Mr. Martin worked with data processing equipment and required manual dexterity in his work. Dr. Bralliar, a surgeon, was consulted. Dr. Bralliar treated Mr. Martin, recommending surgery to repair tendons and put a finger in a functional position. Mr. Martin was concerned about the function of the finger. Dr. Bralliar assured him there would be no problem. Following surgery and removal of the cast, two of Mr. Martin's fingers were curled and he was unable to move them. When the condition did not improve, Dr. Bralliar said it was due to scar tissue and suggested a second operation. This operation produced no change in Mr. Martin's condition. Dr. Bralliar advised an amputation of the fifth finger. The patient sued.

Evidence at the trial revealed that the patient was not informed of any risks involved in the hand surgery. Dr. Bralliar admitted he made the statement that "there should be no problems." At the trial, medical experts testified that immobilization longer than a week for this surgery is improper. It could result in contracture, a known substantial risk. Based on all the evidence, the jury awarded Mr. Martin $60,000 as compensatory damages.

The Court of Appeals of Colorado said that the *informed* consent of the patient must be obtained before surgery is performed. It further stated that the doctor must advise the patient not only in a general way about the risks involved, but also of any substantial or specific risks known to the physician.

Duty to Withhold Information   The courts have also held the physician need not disclose the risks of a procedure if they are commonly considered remote and the procedure itself is simple. The risks also need not be disclosed if the patient specifically says he does not want to be informed, or if the physician in his professional judgment and

5   Martin B. Bralliar, 540 P. 2d 1118 (Colorado App. 1975).

discretion reasonably believes the disclosure of the information is not in the best interests of the patient. In such cases it would be wise for the physician to disclose the appropriate information to the next of kin. That type of disclosure would demonstrate the physician's objective interest in the patient's well-being.

Liability of the Nurse

The court cases involving the issue of informed consent are clear and consistent in placing the responsibility of giving the necessary information to the patient to enable him to make an intelligent decision on the physician. The nurse is not the one performing the operation or medical procedure the patient is about to undergo. The nurse, generally, does not have the necessary information nor does she know what alternative procedures are available for the patient. Nurses should not allow themselves to be placed in the ridiculous position of "witnessing the patient's signature." It is common practice for nurses to have the function of getting the patient to sign the hospital consent form. The nurse, generally, has not been present when the physician presumably gave the necessary instructions and explanations to the patient. The process usually follows this pattern. The nurse asks the patient, "Did your doctor explain about your surgery for tomorrow morning?" If the patient answers in the affirmative, the nurse asks the patient to read and sign the consent form. Although it is probably an act of futility because the nurse has not witnessed that the patient gave an informed consent, there is no liability. If the patient answers the nurse's questions in the negative, then the nurse is obligated to see that the appropriate parties are notified so the patient is given the opportunity to give an informed consent. The nurse could be held personally liable if she knew or should have known the patient was uninformed and did not take remedial measures. The hospital could also be held liable under the doctrine of corporate negligence or respondeat superior if, through its personnel, the hospital knew or had reason to know that physicians or staff personnel are performing procedures without a bona fide consent. The nurse has a professional obligation to protect her employer's interests. Since the hospital has an obligation to see that the patient is informed, the nurse would be decreasing the legal risk to the hospital by informing the physician or others of the patients' needs.

Refusal of Treatment   A competent adult patient has the right to refuse medications, treatment, and other proposed health care. The nurse should respect the patient's right to refuse. It is always good practice to document this refusal. If possible, the nurse should have corroboration of this refusal either by the patient writing his refusal or by a competent witness documenting the event or both.

Consent to Transsexual or Sex-Reassignment Surgery

In 1952 a highly publicized transsexual operation took place in Denmark. The operation resulted in a male, George Jorgensen, becoming a female, Christine Jorgensen. A *transsexual* is defined "as an individual with an obsession to belong to the opposite sex which is not practically reversible by psychological or other medical treatment." [1] Radical surgery is necessary. A *transvestite* is defined as a person who wears clothing appropriate to the opposite sex and who desires to be accepted as a member of the opposite sex. A *homosexual* is defined as an individual sexually attracted by persons of the same sex.

The Johns Hopkins Hospital located in Baltimore, Maryland, has done pioneering work in the area of gender identity. The hospital has developed a protocol for the patient intent on making a sexual change to reasonably assure that the operation will be psychologically and physiologically beneficial to the patient. There are states that have laws which could designate certain acts as illegal and could subject the patient to arrest. In some states certain sexual acts between members of the same sex are illegal, but part of the preoperative treatment is that a selected patient must live in the role of the desired sex to prove his ability to function in that sex. Because of this problem, the state health department in the particular state where the patient is receiving treatment issues an identification card to the patient. This card identifies the patient as having a neuroendocrinological condition. Although the card does not completely prevent the patient's possible prosecution, it demonstrates the medical motivation behind certain activities.

Informed Consent   The type of surgery performed is very complex. There is removal of sexual organs and recreation of the organs of the desired sex. There is hormonal therapy involved. Sterility is inherent in the procedure at the present time. Most physicians and hospitals require the patient to have a close relative also involved in the process to assure the informed consent requirements of the law are met and to

---

1   Presser, C. S.: "Legal Problems Attendant to Sex Reassignment Surgery," The Journal of Legal Medicine, Vol. 5, No. 4 (April, 1977), PP. 17-24.

diminish the risk of litigation. This is not required by state law since every competent adult may consent to his own medical treatment, but it is a superimposed policy of the physician or hospital.

Legal Issues   Transsexuals are advised to change their name in accord with the sex change. The legal procedure for changing the information on a birth certificate varies from state to state. The transsexual should give attention to any other legal or official documents such as wills, passports, licenses, social security and pension benefits which may adversely affect him unless the documents are corrected or amended. There are problems to be anticipated in the area of marriage. Once the transsexual has assumed a new sex, he can not participate in a marriage with a member of the same sex. If the transsexual is presently married, the marriage might become void by operation of law or the operation itself might provide grounds for a divorce depending on the various state statutes.

There is a great amount of time and preparation devoted to pre-operative counseling with the individual undergoing transsexual surgery. It is done both in psychological and anatomical stages. Because of the intense preparation and the absolute involvement of the patient in every phase of care, it is doubtful that a charge of lack of informed consent would be a valid charge under the usual circumstances of transsexual surgery.

Case on Doctrine of Informed Consent
Appellate Court Case
Kruszewski vs. Holz—May 1972

This case involves a suit for alleged malpractice for not informing a patient of alternatives to performance of an operation. The plaintiff was a 47-year-old woman complaining of irregular, frequent, painful, and heavily bleeding menstrual periods. This occurred in the fall of 1967 and Dr. Holz performed dilatation and curettage, a D & C. In May of 1968, the symptoms reappeared along with a small lump on her left breast. Dr. Holz referred Mrs. Kruszewski to a general

Void: having no legal force

2   "Transsexuals in Limbo: The Search for a Legal Definition of Sex," 31 Md. Law Rev. (1971), PP. 236-254. Notes and comments.

surgeon, Dr. Thomas. Dr. Thomas recommended surgery, and if the breast lump was benign, to also do a hysterectomy. Dr. Holz states he warned the patient this was major surgery and complications could arise.

Plaintiff was admitted to the hospital on June 30, 1968 and signed a standard consent form which read in part:

> "The nature and purpose of the operation, possible alternative methods of treatment, the risks involved, and the possibility of complications have been fully explained to me. I acknowledge that no guarantee or assurance has been made as to the result that may be obtained."

On July 1, 1968, the breast growth was removed and a hysterectomy performed. Patient recovered uneventfully and was discharged July 9, 1968. A few days later Mrs. Kruszewski complained of leakage of urine through the vagina and was diagnosed as having a fistula. Patient sued Dr. Holz claiming negligence because 1) he injured the bladder during surgery, and 2) he failed to inform her adequately of the possible risks to the operation.

At issue was the standard of care. The expert witness for the plaintiff, Dr. Harvey Jorgenson, said he believed the defendant doctor did not meet the standard of care normally exercised by physicians because he did not completely inform the patient of all possible complications and risk involved prior to obtaining consent to the hysterectomy. Experts for the defendant, Drs. Dumler and Novak, testified the leakage was due to a thin bladder weakened by the operation. They stated it was *not* standard procedure for a physician in the community to do more than advise the patient that a hysterectomy is major surgery with possible risks and complications.

The jury found for the defendant doctor that he followed the standards of the community when he informed the plaintiff there were possible complications attending hysterectomies. The jury found the doctor was not negligent because he had followed the customary method of informing patients that was followed by competent medical doctors in the area.

There was no elaboration on what should or should not be included in determining informed consents. The court looked at all the circumstances surrounding the consent and determined if in the particular case sufficient information was given for the patient to make an intelligent decision about her operation. The court held sufficient information was given.

INVOLUNTARY COMMITMENT

Mental capacity or *competence* is defined as the ability to understand the nature and effect of the act in which a person is engaged and the business he is transacting.

Mental incapacity or incompetency is established when there is found to exist an essential privation of reasoning faculties, or when a person is incapable of understanding and acting with discretion in the ordinary affairs of life. The terms are more descriptive of certain categorical behaviors rather than definitions. A voluntary admission to a psychiatric health care setting is one where the patient freely consents to be admitted and submit to treatment.

A patient who voluntarily enters such an institution may freely leave at any time without any formalities. An involuntary admission to a psychiatric health care setting is one where the patient is admitted against his will. Each state has certain procedures which must be followed for an involuntary admission of an individual to occur. Involuntary admissions are generally classified as emergency or non-emergency admissions.

Emergency Admission and Non-Emergency Admission

Admission   At common law no individual could be deprived of his liberty and hospitalized against his will unless the individual was an imminent danger to himself or others.

Most states have passed legislation establishing a criteria for emergency hospitalization. The essential criteria is similar from state to state, although there may be variations in procedure and interpretation of the terms of the criteria. The standard or criteria require that the evidence establish that the individual has a mental illness, is imminently dangerous to himself or others, and is in need of institutionalization. The wording in the California, Massachusetts, and Maryland statutes are very clear in defining what is meant by "dangerous to oneself and others."

Procedure   Most states permit emergency commitment of an individual based on the certification of two physicians; the two physicians do not need to be psychiatrists. They must certify that they have personally examined the individual and believe him to be mentally ill and a danger to himself or others.

Due process is a term that connotatively has come to mean "fair play." The United States Constitution mandates that everyone must be given due process of law before any deprivation of liberty can take place. This means essentially that the citizen must be notified of the allegations which are the basis for the proposed deprivation of liberty, that the citizen be given an opportunity to rebut the charges against him, and that the citizen be given an opportunity to be heard by an impartial party who will weigh all sides of the issues. The essence of due process is that every man is entitled to his day in court.

In a non-emergency judicial proceeding, the hearing officer or judge must find as a fact that the individual is mentally ill and a danger to himself or others. If this determination is made, the commitment may be ordered. In an emergency judicial proceeding, the hearing officer or judge must have reasonable grounds to believe that the individual is mentally ill and a danger to himself or others. If based on the evidence presented the judge reasonably concludes the above, then an emergency commitment can be made. This emergency commitment suffices to protect the individual and others for a specific time period until a fuller determination of the need for commitment can be made under less expedient circumstances. This permits a full judicial hearing and necessitates a court order before an involuntary commitment of institutionalization and consequent deprivation of liberty can take place.

Voluntary Admission A *voluntary admission* is one in which an individual freely consents to enter an institution for the purported purpose of needing and receiving psychiatric care and treatment. It is made without undue influence, coercion, or duress. An individual who enters a psychiatric center voluntarily may leave just as any other citizen and may not be held against his will or wishes. The exception would be where the person has entered voluntarily and the psychiatric hospital or center begins involuntary commitment proceedings.

The institutionalized patient can always file a writ of habeas corpus to be released from the hospital.

Periodic Review Most states also require by statute that a periodic review of the institutionalized patient's status be made. The purpose of this statutory provision is to prevent continued unnecessary con-

Allegation: a charge
Habeas Corpus: "to have the body," a petition for release where an individual is unjustly or illegally detained or confined

finement. The review permit varies from state to state, but the average review time is six months to a year.

Right to Treatment   Presumably the psychiatric care concept has made progress since the time of Dorthea Dix (1883–1887), a crusader for the humane care of the mentally ill. As early as 1845, Chief Justice Shaw of the Massachusetts Supreme Court laid down the precedent that individuals could only be restrained if dangerous to themselves or others. Emphasis is on treatment, behavior modification, or rehabilitation of the mentally ill person. The goal of working with mentally ill patients is one of resocialization, having them return to the community at large. The question then is to ask if the institutionalization is offering treatment directed at this goal? If it is, then institutionalization can be justified. If it is not, then how can institutonalization be justified? The era of simply "warehousing" individuals with mental illness is over.

Admission of Minors to Mental Health Care Agencies

In the majority of states, parents may place a child in a psychiatric setting without the child's consent. The deprivation of liberty is just as real as that for an adult, yet there is no equivalent due process protection afforded the juvenile. There is present litigation challenging the lack of procedural protection for the minor. In *Bartley v. Kremens*[1] case, the constitutionality of the Pennsylvania Mental Health and Retardation Act was challenged. The main issue was whether a child's interest in not being institutionalized is protected by the fourteenth amendment. The Federal Court concluded that a child is entitled to the procedural protection of due process and that parents and guardians cannot waive this right. The rights of the child are weighed against the rights of the parents in raising the child. The state has an interest in several parties. It has an interest in preserving the authority of the parent and the family unit as well as in the physical and mental health of the child. It also has an interest in protecting society at large from the potential danger of injurious activity by children with mental disorders.

Due Process: certain procedural requirements to assure fairness

[1]   *Bartley v. Kremens*, 402 F. Supp. 1039 (E.D. Pa. 1975), Prob. Juris. Noted, 96 S. Ct. 1457 (1976).

The courts are concerned that where a conflict between the child's interest and the parents' interest exists, there is some independent authority to evaluate the child's need for institutionalization. A classical example of parent-child conflict is child abuse. There are also times when parents resolve other conflicts with the child by admitting the child to a mental institution. Anyone who has had contact with mental institutions is aware that admission to an instituion is not necessarily assurance of therapeutic treatment.

CONFIDENTIALITY

Definition of Privacy

The law has always attempted to protect the individual citizen's right to be free from unwarranted intrusion into his private life. A review of the legal and philosophical literature reveals that there is no common definition of privacy. Some perceive privacy as a psychological state of being apart from others. Some perceive privacy as the power to control information about their lives. Others see privacy as the freedom not to participate in the activities of others. Therefore, the fourth amendment right to constitutional justifiable expectations of privacy is subject to diverse definitions.

The best definition appears to be the composite list presented at the International Commission of Justice in 1970. *Privacy* is the ability to lead one's life without anyone: A) interfering with his family and home life; B) interfering with his physical or mental integrity or his moral and intellectual freedom; C) attacking his honor and reputation; D) placing him in a false light; E) disclosing irrelevant embarrassing facts about him; F) misusing his private communications, written or oral; and G) disclosing information given or received in circumstances of professional confidence.[1]

The common law of the right to privacy protection began in 1890 with a law review article by Louis Brandeis, a legal scholar. In it, Brandeis called for a doctrine of privacy per se and the right to be let alone. The Restatement of Torts, Section 652A, recognizes a tort for invasion of privacy where there has been unreasonable intrusion on the seclusion of another or unreasonable publicity given to one's private life or publicity which unreasonably places another in a false public light.

---

[1] Conclusion of the Nordic Conference on the Right of Privacy, *Privacy and the Law*, A Report by the British Section of the International Commission of Justice 45 (Littman and Carter-Ruchens, 1970).

There is an assumption in business and government that individual privacy must yield to the greater social benefits to be gained by the use of information about private individuals. So we find the pervading contention—the individual's right to privacy of personal data is outweighed by society's right to know; generally, the courts agree. The courts generally find that a legitimate business or government interest is one of conditional privilege, and unless there is a showing of malice or that parties without legitimate interest had access to individual's data, the courts deny relief. Therefore, in the absence of malice or illegitimate disclosure, generally the individual has no cause of action against the reporting agency. Legal scholars, some of whom are justices of the Supreme Court, advocate a clearer definition and understanding of what privacy entails.

Right of Privacy

The right of privacy is the right of the individual to be let alone. To be free from unwarranted publicity and public view is a right recognized by law. To live without your name, picture, or private affairs being made public without your consent is also a right. The health care professional cannot divulge information regarding a patient and may be liable for revealing personal information about a patient without the patient's permission or without statutory authority. But the patient may authorize the release of his medical information.

When the patient consents to release of information, the consent must be free, voluntary, and unambiguous. It should also be an informed consent in each and every circumstance. The standard to be applied is that of reasonableness. In order to validly consent, one must understand what the consent involves. A person who is not given sufficient facts cannot make an intelligent decision. The term *sufficient* is used because it would be impossible or unreasonable to expect every fact to be available to the patient before a decision.

In general, consent means voluntary submission. Where the medical record of the patient is involved, any personal, confidential information pertaining to the patient should not be released without his voluntary approval. Oral consent is as valid and binding as written consent. If there were a question of potential litigation, the written consent would be tangible evidence of at least voluntary submission.

Data Handlers As a universally moral precept and legal responsibility, it should be well understood that anyone who handles personal, confidential information for a patient or anyone else is a data handler and owes a duty of care to the protection of the information. The data handlers also have a responsibility to be certain that information is accurate, relevant, current, and secure against any abuse.

The increase in persons, agencies, and third party payors or third parties of miscellaneous nature who have a legitimate interest in a person's medical record has expanded beyond the simple patient, doctor, hospital triangle of yesteryear's era. The problem of maintaining and protecting the patient's privacy has increased proportionately.

The data in a medical record can be classified as *informational* and *clinical* or *confidential* and *non-confidential*. *Informational data* gives certain data such as where patient works, name of insurer, age and marital status. The *clinical data* refers to the diagnosis, treatment and progress of the medical or clinical aspect of patient's care. The *confidential data* is that data of a personal and private nature generally found in the clinical part of the record.[2]

The *non-confidential* data generally relates to identification of the specific patient. Quite often it is the same as the informational data; for example, name, address, age, admission date, discharge date, and certain statistical information. Although non-confidential data can be released without written consent of the patient, it should be done with care. The hospital or agency should have clearly defined policies and procedures on what may be disclosed and by whom. There should be an appropriate person named to be contacted if there is any doubt about disclosure. A conservative policy of releasing information is always recommended.

Confidential Nature of Health Information Data   Health professionals dealing with patient information know or should know that they have a responsibility of not disclosing private information about patients. The ethical standards of the health professionals are extended to all personnel handling patient information, such as data processing persons.

The medical record (that is, the physical property itself) belongs to the health agency or institution. The contents of the record "belong" to several parties, meaning that these parties have the right to have access to the information or the right to have specific sections of the medical record disclosed to them.

Any custodian of medical information—hospital, health agency, doctor—must be continuously aware of the private and confidential nature of the health-related information received. There is a trend to allow the patient to see his record at any reasonable time. The trend is developing nationally and many states permit the patient or his

2   Springer, Eric, *Automated Medical Records and the Law*, P. 62.

authorized agent to examine the medical record at reasonable and appropriate times. The patient always has a right to petition the court to see his record, but as a practical matter, court intervention only arises in cases involving litigation and not merely to review one's medical record as a point of information.

Some authorities claim that hospital records are comparable to public records and should be available to anyone who can demonstrate a legitimate interest or need to have access to the information. There are times when a state statute mandates certain records be made accessible to agencies who do not have direct care or interest in the patient. For example, as a result of increasing malpractice litigation, some legislatures have passed a law commanding malpractice insurance agencies to give all requested information to the commission on medical discipline.[3] The information generally pertained to physicians who were sued for malpractice and negotiated settlements which were not matters of public record.

Permissable Disclosure of Medical Information

The principal consideration in disclosure in absence of the patient's authorization is the legitimate interest of the person or agencies and the nature of the health or related data requested.

Hospitals and health agencies should establish policies and procedures relating to disclosure of information to parties not connected with the health agency by employment or association. These policies and procedures should recognize the responsibilities to patients and legitimate interest of third party payors, researchers, attorneys, and the press. Procedures should be followed to assure that only authorized persons will have access to the medical information and only authorized requests will be processed.

Parties Generally Having Legitimate Interest   All persons involved in the direct or indirect health care of a patient would be considered as having a legitimate interest. Insurance companies or third party payors are recognized as having a legitimate interest in the patient's record. There is an administrative procedure to be followed before insurance companies will assure payment; and patients and health agencies recognize this. Attorneys may obtain the patient's record if the patient gives written authorization.

3   *Bader v. United Orthodox Synagogue*, 172 A2d 192.

Governmental Agencies   The majority of legal experts advise that a health agency should cooperate with bona fide representatives of governmental agencies such as law enforcement, Veteran's Administration, state coroner's office. Certain agencies are given expressed legislative authority to obtain medical record information if there is a legitimate public interest. There are occasions when there is a legal duty to disclose information; for example, cases involving gunshot wounds, child abuse, communicable diseases, and venereal disease. In such instances, the appropriate public or health officials should be notified.

News Media   The news media has a legitimate interest in patient information where the newsworthiness of a particular event outweighs the right to privacy. There are times when a news event may be disclosed without consent or authorization. Discretion and good business dictates that release of information to reporters should be prepared by a public relations person. It is further suggested that the public relations officer prepare the statement in conjunction with the physician, medical record librarian, and administrator. There are exceptions to the right of privacy, such as when the public's right to know outweighs the individual's right to privacy. The actions of a public person are of legitimate interest to the public and the news media has a right to report them. The media has a right to report and photograph the subjects of a newsworthy event.

Personnel   Personnel handling confidential information should be required to take appropriate courses in understanding the nature and confidentiality of the data they handle. The course should cover the ethical, professional, and legal responsibilities of the data handled. The personnel should have access to policies and procedures which govern the flow of information to individuals and health agencies and other parties having a legitimate interest. The policies and procedures should be developed by the interdisciplinary committee and all employees should be kept currently informed of policy. The personnel should know the protective procedures to safeguard and prevent inadvertent disclosure of confidential information.

Liability for Disclosure of Confidential Information

The issue of liability in releasing data of a private nature from a patient's record is of concern to health care providers.

There are two broad areas of liability to be considered. The first is liability for unwarranted or unauthorized disclosure. Where confidential information is revealed by the hospital or health care agency and the patient proves damages, the patient may sue on the theory of defamation or invasion of privacy. Where a health professional has disclosed confidential information, the patient may seek relief as above and may report the professional to the appropriate professional society for censure or to the appropriate licensing body for a hearing to challenge the practitioner's right to practice his profession. When that duty is breached, the liability attaches directly to the hospital or agency.

Although the hospital or health agency as an entity does not practice medicine, it can be vicariously liable for the acts of its employees under the doctrine of respondeat superior (let the master respond). It is based on the fact that the employer has the right to control the employee's performance, and therefore is responsible for the actions of the employee. The employer is obligated to control the employee in protecting the patient's privacy.

In order to sue successfully for defamation, libel, and slander, it is necessary to show that the disclosure of confidential medical information was both unauthorized and untrue. Most data collected in medical records is factual material. Since truth is a complete defense to a charge of defamation there is limited risk that a lawsuit would be successful based on these circumstances.

Of more concern is litigation based on the theory of invasion of privacy. The theory is that patients are entitled to be free of unwarranted disclosures of personal information, even if the disclosed information is true. A cause of action could arise from the unauthorized disclosure of medical record information if the information would be of such a nature as to offend a person of ordinary sensibilities. Generally, hospital or health data is not sufficiently offensive to be actionable.

A potential area for a lawsuit for invasion of privacy is disclosure of unauthorized information to insurance companies. In a 1965 case, *Hammonds v. Aetna Casualty and Surety Company* (243 F. Supp. 793), Aetna Casualty was sued by Hammonds because the insurance company induced a physician to reveal confidential medical information. The Ohio court, ruling in favor of Hammonds, said there was a legal and ethical duty to keep patient information confidential and the physician breached that duty.

In *Horne v. Patton* (287 Sa. 2d 824), a 1973 Alabama case, a doctor revealed medical data to a patient's employer without authorization, resulting in termination of the job of the patient-employee.

The court held that an employer does not necessarily have a legitimate interest in an employee's health history.

The fear of litigation makes custodians of medical records cautious. The release of confidential information is based on: 1) the authorization of the patient; 2) the judicial mandate; and 3) statutory mandate, such as reporting communicable disease or child abuse.

Interchange of Confidential Information between Professional Health Persons or Agencies   The general public's acceptance of the computer as a factor in their everyday life is reflected in present banking and business procedures. Today when we purchase clothes at the department store or food at a supermarket, the "magic buttons" quickly assume responsibility for the transaction. But the ingenuity does not stop at the counter; the computer follows through to alert the appropriate parties that there has been a decrease in the inventory and prepares a statement for restocking. The implementation of sophisticated automation in the medical field is in the embryonic stage as far as the true potential for its uses. Few of us can envision what uses will be devised for the computer in the health care delivery system by the year 2000.

There is a very real *caveat* or warning to all who are contemplating the use of computers in collection of patient information. The caveat of confidentiality with all the legal ramifications is given repeatedly in the literature on the topic of computerized medical records. At the same time, the potential for increasing quality care, decreasing cost, and decreasing legal liability is one of the strongest reasons for moving quickly to using computerized data systems.

The question of confidentiality, invasion of privacy, and physician patient privileged communication are basic questions that go to the fiduciary relationships all health professionals owe to their client, the patient. Whether manual or computerized, whether for medical or for business purposes, the basic element in the system is respect and appreciation of the individual's right to privacy.

A patient places the integrity of his person and reputation in the hands of the health care personnel when he submits himself to their care. The inviolability of the patient's privacy is protected by law and public policy. It is considered to be in the public interest that persons seeking treatment or therapy be protected from public exposure due to confidential or personal information being disclosed.

Although we have inherited much of our law from the common law of England, there was no right of confidentiality or patient privilege at common law. The right of privacy and confidentiality is a creature of statutory law enacted by the states.

Distinction Between Confidential Communication and Privileged Communication

There is an important distinction between confidential communications and privileged communications. A *confidential communication* is a communication made by a patient to a health care practitioner in the course of caring for that patient. It is information entrusted to the health care practitioner that should not be revealed except in certain circumstances. It is considered a breach of professional ethics for any health care practitioner to repeat or reveal any information about a patient. In certain states laws have been enacted called *privileged communication statutes.* These laws provide that certain categories of persons, that is, attorney-client, psychiatrist-patient, and priest-penitent, have a special privilege. The special privilege is that the information received by the special categories of persons cannot be forced to be revealed in any legal proceedings without the specific consent of the client, patient or penitent or any other category of persons specified in the statute. Where the communication is confidential and not privileged, the court may, in appropriate cases, order the communication to be revealed in testimony.

In regard to the health care area, the privileged communication of the patient extends to written communications such as the medical record as well as oral statements. The patient's consent should be obtained before revealing any confidential information about the patient.

There are certain government agencies who have not only the right but the mandated duty to collect normally confidential, private information. Such agencies are the Internal Revenue Service, The Department of Labor, The Environmental Protection Agency, and The Equal Employment Office. Some of this information may be transmitted from agency to agency depending on the authority of the agency, the relationship, and the sanctions provided according to the law.[4]

Access to Records   The patient has a fiduciary relationship with hospitals, doctors, health agencies, and health care workers. The cus-

Fiduciary: trust

[4]   Privacy. *Practising Law Institute,* 1974, Volume 1970.

todian of the patient's personal data must be cognizant of the confidential nature of the information received during patient care. The patient can authorize his attorney to procure the medical records and thus circumvent a refusal by administrators for the patient to see the records. And, of course, any court can issue the order known as *subpoena duces tecum* ("bring the documents") and it would have to be obeyed. The majority opinion is that the patient should be entitled to full disclosure of his record. The question is: Why should health professionals, review committees, insurers, government agencies, and researchers have access and not the patient?

The Secretary's Commission on Medical Malpractice stated that the patient has a right to the information contained in the medical record.[5] This statement by the commission carries no legal mandate, but it will hopefully influence the trend to inform patients more fully. It is ironic that in most jurisdictions the patient can authorize attorneys, insurance companies, doctors, and other "appropriate" persons to see his medical record but cannot have direct access to them himself.

Summary

The questions of confidentiality, invasion of privacy, and privileged communications are basic questions that go to the fiduciary relationships all health care professionals owe to their client, the patient. The basic element in any communications system, whether oral or written, is respect for the individual's right to privacy. A patient places the integrity of his person and reputation in the hands of the health care practitioner when he submits himself to their care. The inviolability of the patient's privacy is protected by law and public policy. The integrity of the confidentiality of the health care system is directly related to the integrity of the personnel, professional and non-professional, who function in the system.

MEDICAL RECORDS

The medical record of a patient is a written account of what has happened to that patient during a special time. This happening can occur in a doctor's office, a hospital, a nursing home, health maintenance organization, or any place in which medical care is given. It is, there-

5 Curran, William J. et. al., "Protection of Privacy and Confidentiality," *Science*, Volume 182 (November, 1973).

fore, a business record and as such is admissible into the appropriate court as evidence. The medical record serves many functions. One main function is as a source of accurate communication between health professionals and other legitimate or appropriate persons or agencies. The medical record has taken on new dimensions because of medical audit, peer review, utilization review, infection control and other tangential areas affected by federal and state legislation and hospital licensing and accreditation requirements. The uses for the patient's medical record are not yet fully realized because changes in technology, legislation, and consumer demands have demonstrated new roles for it.

The medical record is an official document. It is a document which quite often is utilized to resolve controversial issues. The medical record of almost every patient will be involved in third party payments, personal injury cases, disability claims, workmen's compensation, insurance and medical negligence cases. It is a confidential document and is the physical property of the hospital. The hospital is the official repository of the medical record.

Some purposes of the medical record are to:

1. Provide a means of communication for health professionals caring for patients;
2. Serve as data basis for planning individual care and clinical data for research or education and unanticipated future events;
3. Serve as statistical information for public health care data and state planning agencies;
4. Be of use to the Joint Commission on Accreditation of Hospitals and state planning agencies for evaluation and accreditation;
5. Serve as documentary evidence for patient for workmen's compensation, pension, insurance, and in the event of litigation; and
6. Serve as an objective witness to certain events that occurred in a health care setting.

The medical record system is required to contain sufficient information to justify the diagnosis, course, management, and treatment of the patient. That information should be accurate, secure, objective, and reliable. The rationale for treatment of the patient is based on the conclusions reached by analyzing and correlating all the information in the record.

In reviewing the purpose of the medical record, little, if any, attention has been given to the iatrogenic effect of medicine and the relation to accurate and complete information. In the late 1930's, irradiation was commonly prescribed for certain throat and skin conditions. It was an effective and relatively inexpensive treatment. However, evidence began to accumulate in the early 1950's that irradiation was carcinogenic. Several incidents of thyroid cancer were identified and in July of 1973, DeGrout and Paloyan were able to scientifically establish a direct link between the irradiation procedure and cancer of the thyroid. Fortunately, this particular cancer is a slow growing tumor and is responsive to treatment.

When this information was made available to hospitals, physicians and health care agencies, the reaction was an ambivalent one. Some institutions elected not to do anything fearing a triggering of malpractice suits. Some institutions had not kept records which could identify potential victims and had no ability to locate them.

The main investigative tool was the medical record. The awesome question of who shall live or who shall die was dependent on the adequacy of content written 10, 20, 30 years before, without the realization of iatrogenesis. The word itself was unknown at that time.

If this and similar types of studies covering a variety of health states are validated, what is the implication for the medical record?

Nurses Notes

Nurses are often quoted as saying, "Why should we write notes?" "They are unimportant." "No one ever reads them." "They are not kept as a permanent part of the record." . . . Do not accept these statements. Many a court case has been won or lost on the nurses' notes in the chart. The nurses' notes in the *Nork* case became critical to ascertaining the truth. (See reference to *Nork* case in corporate negligence, page 33.)

The medical record should be a document which describes the patient's medical event in a systematic, organized manner, including patient's problems, reactions and responses to procedures, medications, diet, and treatment. If the patient complains of pain, the notes should indicate where the pain is located, severity of it, what it is associated with, for example, diet, getting into or out of bed, post surgery, x-ray, or operation. If medication is given, anything resulting from the medication should be noted. Instead of saying, "patient appears weak," the notes should state "cannot walk without assistance" or "cannot sip fluid through straw."

Iatrogenesis: medically induced

The medical record should be able to identify and provide necessary information to notify patients who have been treated or medicated that an iatrogenic effect or technological advancement presently indicates a danger to their health and perhaps their life. Should a cure or palliative measure be available, it should be made immediately obtainable to the patients involved. The health care professional has a new consideration in keeping medical records. There should be sufficient identifying information about the treatments and procedures performed on a patient to enable an investigator to make a proper judgment and take steps to initiate corrective measures where there is potential iatrogenic illness.

If you initiate care or perform a procedure on the basis of standing orders, you should be certain to identify the signs, symptoms, and any other indications for your action. This is for your own best interest. Your first duty is to yourself. Therefore, you should indicate the basis and reasons for your decisions to implement standing orders. Another method of notation is to correlate what you see with what you know. For example, if the patient is bleeding the first time you see him and you take his pulse, the next time you take that pulse indicate if stronger or weaker beat. This is a subjective symptom but the same person is making the comparison; therefore, the subjectivity has a standard against which it is being measured.

If the patient complains of nausea and vomiting, blurred vision, rash, or other symptoms, the nurse should review medications because many hospitals separate notes from medication sheets and relationships are often not established. A patient is often treated for a condition without the cause being ascertained. Drug interaction could be the etiological factor and often the obvious is overlooked.

In general, nurses' notes should reflect factual information: what you see—drainage, what kind, color, amount; what you feel—lump, what kind, size, consistency (that is, what your senses perceive); what you do for the patient; what the response is to your actions. If policy indicates specific action such as use of bed rails, restraints, or wheelchair, indicate what was done and why.

Attempting to convince a jury that you did a particular action several years earlier that is not substantiated in the chart may stretch the credulity of the jury in convincing them that you remember details of a particular patient's care.

Never is the maxim, "We never have time to do it right the first time, but we always have time to do it over again" more true than with medical records. It is better to write correct notes than to answer questions years later on the lack of information in your chart.

One way to keep out of court is to write a complete and honest report. Fully describe the situation by giving the hospital attorney enough information so he can make a judgment about recommending settlement or non-settlement, or preparing and pursuing a proper defense in court.

Probably the most common error in hospital records and one which decreases the value of the record is reporting value judgments, opinion, conjectures, and conclusions instead of factual observations. For example, in an emergency room notation do not write, "appears to have fractured right arm." Proper notation would be, "has bruised area two cm in size, scratches on right arm and other signs of injury." It is up to other appropriate parties to draw inferences and make conclusions. An entry "it appears that" does not make a fact out of a conclusion. That type of introduction weakens the fact; it indicates the writer was uncertain, or unsure of his own perceptions. Notes or incidents charted should relate specifically to care of patient. For example, color, temperature, pulse, blanching of part involved, medication—what reaction, if any. You should be like an investigator; present facts, not conclusions. Give objective statements, not commentary. Let the reader draw the conclusion.

Legally, the medical record is important in a malpractice suit. It can be subpoenaed and brought to court. The data in the record can make or break the case.

It should be understood that the individual making notations on the medical record is neither an adversary nor an advocate for the medical record. The role of the notator is that of an objective witness, one who receives certain perceptions through the senses and reports those sensations without embellishment.

Medical records are evidence of certain events. The original entries are made concommitantly with a particular event and with the personal knowledge of the individual delivering or responsible for certain phases of health care. They are not self-authenticating documents and are not made under oath nor are the records subject to cross-examination. The judicial process requires notations be accurate, complete, recorded at the time event took place, without a vested interest, and recorded for professional purposes and not for judicial proceedings. There is a presumption in law that they are true statements. This is a rebuttable presumption.

It is essential that the patient's name be correctly spelled. An incorrect name could infer that improper attention was given to the patient. Correct patient identification is basic to conveying accurate information.

The method of admission to the hospital is important, for example, stretcher, ambulatory, wheelchair, or ambulance. The record should show patient's condition on admission, vital signs, complaints made by patient, time patient was admitted to surgery, x-ray, and time patient left area. This requirement may appear routine and unimportant but can cause grief in later litigation when a critical question arises regarding the patient's ability to ambulate at certain times.

Countersigning   Nursing aides or assistants often perform certain patient tasks but are not permitted to chart the results of their findings. Instead, the aides convey the results to a nurse who charts what has been told to her. The nurse often has no personal knowledge of what she is writing. Frequently she has not seen the patient or the test result and yet she is attesting to the authenticity of events to which she has not been a party.

Anyone who signs a document is presumed to have read the document, and if one places his signature under treatments, medications, and notes, it is presumed that the signer has personal knowledge of the information or performed the particular procedure. Therefore, it is incumbent on anyone who purports to give information on a medical record to know that the information is accurate. Therefore, if your signature appears on the record in a capacity other than having personal knowledge of the particular events, explain the capacity clearly so that in the event of litigation, your position is not misconstrued. For example, if the handling of the record is for review and medical audit, then the signatory should make that clear to the reader.

There are institutions who use check lists to conserve time in conveying information. There is nothing improper in using check lists. The question is, does the check list supply all the relevant and necessary information to make a judgment about the patient's case based on that information? If the answer is no, the health care practitioner should supplement the check list with an addendum, adding any material information that is significant in the case of the patient.

Handlers of medical records often construe the format of the medical record as sacrosanct and hesitate to add anything to a particular form. If it is necessary to add a sentence or even a page to clarify the facts and to protect yourself legally, then do so. Brevity is a commendable attribute, but the essence of effective documentation is the presentation of all the facts. Essential, factual information should never be sacrificed in the interest of brevity. The authors are not advocating disregard of form but want to emphasize the need for clarifi-

Signatory: one who signs
Sacrosanct: not to be violated

cation regardless of format. Persons who give the service should initial
or sign for that service. A registered nurse or licensed practical nurse
should not sign or initial for care given by another person. To have
the record show that the nurse gave service which she did not give is
a disservice to the patient. The nurse and the hospital could be liable
for actions that border on fraud or misrepresentation. If the registered
nurse is responsible for checking a patient's record and signing it, the
signature should show that is what was done by noting, "checked the
record and signed it."

The written document would outweigh the oral disclaimer of
"that wasn't the way it happened." Plus, will you recall five, six, or
ten years later who gave a particular service and under what circumstances? In general, the health care practitioner should write only
information on the chart which he knows from his own first-hand
observations, or which he has validated as accurate.

Remember, to *countersign* by definition, is "to place one's signature to a writing already signed by another to attest to the authenticity
of that writing." If your reason for countersigning is not compatible
with the definition, it would be judicious to analyze and review your
purpose before committing yourself to possible legal risk.

Alteration

Records which have been altered for any reason, however innocent or pragmatic, should always include notations of the date, reason
for change and initials, or signature and position of person altering
the record. If a negligence suit is filed subsequent to a record being
altered, it could well be construed as an attempt to avoid liability or
to deliberately mislead the court. If alteration was dishonestly made,
it could well result in a criminal charge of obstructing justice or
fraudulent misrepresentation.

Obviously one should never erase anything on a patient's record.
An erasure raises questions and is equivalent to telling the jury you
are hiding something. If an entry is erroneous, clearly draw a line
through the error, write "error" to the side in parentheses, enter the
correction, add your signature and the date. If explanation seems appropriate, give it; forms are not sacrosanct. Do not hesitate to clarify
or explain the reason for the situation. In certain risky situations, it is
prudent to have your corrected notation witnessed by a co-worker.

There is another type of alteration that must be considered. It is
the situation where the administrator calls a nurse into his office and
states that Dr. Wampum Donor has complained about the nurses' notes

on the chart not being accurate or being improper observations. The doctor wants them changed or removed from the chart. Parenthetically it is noted that Dr. Wampum Donor is one of the biggest contributors to the building fund. This is not a hypothetical case. It has happened and does continue to happen. Anyone who would submit to this kind of pressure is placing himself in the worst of legal positions. He could be guilty of malpractice and also of fraud, misrepresentation, and possibly a criminal charge of obstruction of justice. Each professional must write his notes from his own vantage point. It is quite conceivable that there could be a contradiction in physician's notes and nurse's notes. This does not necessarily mean a conflict and confrontation must follow. The courts recognize that reasonable men differ in their perceptions of a particular event. Let each participant in health care document their own observations according to their own insights.

Access to Medical Records

What rights, if any, does a patient have to his medical records?

Hospital records (that is the physical property itself) are normally the property of the hospital, but the content of those records can be inspected and copied at appropriate times by a patient's legal guardian or his attorney with written permission of the patient. In some states the patient does not have the right to read his records but in all states the patient's attorney has the right of access. If a doctor or hospital unjustifiably refuses access to those records, a charge of *fraudulent concealment* might result in the statute of limitations being extended to sue from the time the records are made available to the patient's representative.

Medical records, such as admission lists, change of shift memos, or surgical logbooks which refer to groups of patients, might not be subject to access. But the courts have allowed a patient access to that portion of the document which is relevant to or specifically refers to the patient.

Medical records are often replete with the third party statements. It is customary for recorders of hospital events to write what has been told to them by a party other than the patient. For example, a nursing aide will report to the charge nurse that a patient is complaining of pain in the abdomen. The charge nurse in turn will tell the medication nurse to initiate alleviating the patient's pain. The charge nurse may write on the patient's chart, "complaining of pain," yet has never seen the patient. The validation of the patient's complaint has never taken place. The charge nurse does not have first hand, direct knowledge of the event she is recording. Normally courts would not admit into evidence such "hearsay evidence."

The medical record, however, is an exception. Under the Uniform Business Records as Evidence Act, hospital records relating to the subject being adjudicated are admissible. The court assumes the information is made in the ordinary course of hospital business and without vested interest.

Generally, governmental agencies have no right to inspect the medical records of a patient without a court order. Medical records should not be released to social or investigatory agencies without the consent of the patient or a court order, unless there is a statutory requirement clearly integrated into hospital policy with appropriate procedures and guidelines to be followed before release of any information.

Length of Time Records are Retained The minimal amount of time records should be kept is at least the number indicated in the statute of limitations. In the instance of a minor patient, records should be kept until the age of majority (18 or 21 years) plus the statute of limitations allowing a minor to bring suit for injuries sustained during minority. The optimal retention is to make all patient records permanent records. As indicated previously, iatrogenic factors and other unanticipated events make it more necessary than ever before to recognize that medical records are as significant as birth or death certificates and more important for daily functioning.

Summary

Although the medical record is used in many controversial issues, the value of properly maintaining the quality, relevancy, objectivity, and accuracy of the medical record is uncontroverted. The responsibility for this maintenance rests with all health care professionals.

In this century, medical records have become interrelated in every aspect of health care. Every major task or issue in the health care field either begins or ends with the medical record. Medical records should provide substantive and substantiated facts as evidenced by skilled personnel who analyze the quality of care given and the basic reasons for the choice of care. Like any witness, the medical record can be adversary or advocate. If properly written and maintained, the record will be your primary defense witness and your advocate in any official proceeding.

BIBLIOGRAPHY

1. "History of Medical Record Science," *Medical Record News,* October, 1969, Volume 40, No. 5.
2. "What You Haven't Read About the Nork Case," *Medical Economics,* July 22, 1974.
3. Addenbrooke, Dr. F. Clarke, Letter: "Confidentiality of Medical Records," *British Medical Journal,* 1 (5948): 39, January 4, 1975.
3A. Bush, Vanessa, "New Data Battle: State's Need to Know vs. Patient's Privacy," *Modern Health Care,* May, 1975.
4. Curran, W. J., E. M. Laska, H. Kaplan, R. Bank, "Protection of Privacy and Confidentiality, *Science,* 182 (114): 797-892, November, 1973.
5. Accreditation Manual for Hospitals, Joint Commission on Hospital Accreditation, Chicago, Illinois, December, 1970.
6. Karst, Kenneth L., "The Files," Legal Control Over the Accuracy and Accessibility of Stored Personal Data, Professor of Law, University of California, Los Angeles.

Also:

Report of the Secretary's Advisory Committee on Automated Personal Data Systems. *Records Computers and the Rights of Citizens.* Department of Health, Education and Welfare Publication, July, 1973.

Report of the Secretary's Commission on Medical Malpractice. Washington, D.C. Department of Health, Education and Welfare, No. (05) 73-88, 1973.

Part Three
VIGNETTES

INTRODUCTION TO VIGNETTES

The vignettes presented in Part Three of this text represent actual work situations. These situations were collected over a two-year period from health care practitioners across the United States. The material was correlated for common denominators and the vignettes are the result.

There was repeated concern over the issues of informed consent, restraints, resuscitation, verbal orders, scope of practice, confidentiality, staffing shortages, responsibility for peers or other co-workers, and assuming pharmacy responsibilities. These issues formed the core for the development of the specific situations with suggested answers. Other situations developed that were of sufficient concern and current interest to warrant incorporation. The individual vignettes were developed to cover different subjects in various categories within the health care field. Answers without the understanding of basic principles of law would defeat the purpose of the text.

To understand the concepts of law is a challenging endeavor. The dynamics of law result in different outcomes in cases depending on the application of principles, the facts and circumstances of each situation.

The variety of vignettes is presented as a method of permitting the reader to apply the knowledge learned in previous chapters. The authors are aware that sufficient information necessary to answer the vignettes thoroughly was not covered in the preceding chapters. It would take several volumes of law to assure that all topics were adequately covered. But basic legal information and concepts have been given. The issues presented by the vignettes are situations and problems presented by health practitioners in various states across the nation. There has developed a consensus of problems or questions which resulted in the 32 vignettes which follow. There are some vignettes which have more elaborate answers than others. The reason for this action is that the authors felt the better approach to learning the content was to present the situation and give the answer based on an elaboration of the law, how it is applied in the particular situation, and what implications could result.

Health care practitioners are accustomed to this clinical type of learning process. The abstract concept of sterile technique is taught in the classrooms. The application of that abstraction is developed in the clinical area when doing treatments and procedures.

The vignettes are based on specific legal problems encountered by health practitioners or on the decision of a specific court case. The situation is presented with several questions asked. The reader is requested to act as a jury and make a decision, then answer the questions presented. What judgment or conclusion would you make based on the facts given? What is the rationale in making the particular decision? Some guidelines to assist you in clarifying the facts and coming to a decision are presented following the vignette sequence. The solution or decision recommended by the authors follows the specific vignette on a separate page.

The authors suggest the reader write his answers on a piece of paper prior to reviewing the solution. It is important that the reader does not approach the task conceiving himself as an amateur lawyer and attempting to use a lot of legalese. Rather the reader should understand that the approach is one of developing new concepts, new skills, and learning both to raise questions and to apply learned content to diminish legal risk. One of the most important features of the vignettes is to raise other questions, stimulate the reader to think in more comprehensive legal terms and appreciate the implications and legal consequences of his action. The authors intend for the vignettes to correlate theoretic concepts with contemporary working situations and to assist the reader to develop the "tools" necessary to handle similar situations in his personal life.

VIGNETTE 1

CONFIDENTIALITY AND COMPUTER INFORMATION DATA

Jessie Jetsi was a 73-year-old male patient recuperating from a cerebrovascular accident. Sara Gampie, R.N., was the staff nurse on the unit where Mr. Jetsi had been a patient for three weeks. Mr. Jetsi was making good progress physically, in that he was now able to walk with the aid of a cane and a special arm strap for his partially paralyzed left arm. However, his mental capacity was impaired, and he had a tendency to wander around the unit at times opening doors and closets and acting like a three-year-old child. Dr. Hippo Crate had written an order to have Mr. Jetsi transferred from Healing Arts Hospital to Happy Acres Nursing Home.

Sara Gampie, R.N., called the nursing home and spoke with Clara Bartonette, R.N., nurse in charge of patient admissions. She informed Clara Bartonette that Jessie Jetsi was on his way over via ambulance and should be arriving in 15 minutes. Clara Bartonette requested Sara Gampie to send any and all medical records with Mr. Jetsi so the staff at Happy Acres could plan appropriate care and fill out the nursing care plan. Sara Gampie was very polite and told Clara Bartonette she would like to cooperate with her but could not give or send the requested information. Sara Gampie said Healing Arts Hospital was a very private non-profit institution and would be liable for an invasion of privacy action if they sent Mr. Jetsi's medical records. She could not give any information over the phone because all communications made by the patient to her as a professional nurse were confidential. She felt she was obligated not to reveal any information received under the circumstances. Sara Gampie also stated that most of the information was on computer and automated data process and therefore an even higher degree of confidentiality was required. Clara Bartonette replied by saying, "I need information to institute appropriate care for Mr. Jetsi. You're going to be liable if you don't give me the information."

What, if anything, should Sara Gampie do?
What are the legal implications of the action or inaction on Sara Gampie's part?
What, if any, action should Clara Bartonette take?

Answer

Health care facilities are charged with the responsibility of continuity of care. Therefore, no patient should suffer because of being moved from one facility to another. There should be sufficient and adequate information transmitted with the patient to insure continuity of care. The patient's medical record serves many functions. One primary function is to serve as a source of accurate communication between health professionals and other legitimate or appropriate persons or agencies.

A transfer agreement between the particular health care centers involved in transferring patients would be a preferred arrangement. Such an agreement could specify that there shall be an interchange of certain medical and other information determined to be necessary or useful in the continuity of care of the patient transferred.

The patient should be informed of the need to share certain information with other persons and agencies and sign the appropriate consent form. The release of confidential information is based on: 1) the authorization or consent of the patient; 2) the judicial mandate of the court; and 3) the statutory mandate, such as reporting communicable disease or child abuse.

Many states have regulations implemented as part of the licensing requirements authorizing appropriate exchange of information to insure continuity of care—for example, a patient being transferred from an intermediate care facility to an acute general or special hospital. Obviously, it would be necessary for the receiving institution to have access to the patient's medical information to assure safe and effective continuity of care. It is termed "a need to know" basis.

There is a necessity for balance in the issue of exchange of information as in other legal issues. The balance must be met. An environment must be present where confidentiality and privacy of patient information is respected. Health professionals in all phases and at all levels must be educated and trained to have professional responsibility toward the health care data they handle. It should be understood that exchange of patient information between health care centers does not diminish any of the requirements of the law to protect the patient's privacy. Any unnecessary or inappropriate revelations regarding the patient's condition or situation without appropriate authorization could subject the individual revealing the information to a lawsuit for invasion of privacy, or possible liability or slander, depending on the facts of the situation and the type of information revealed.

VIGNETTE 2

MEDICATION REFUSAL

Mr. Carl Crackers is a 30-year-old male. He is considered to be an exceptional salesman working for Medical Electronics Incorporated. Recently Mr. Crackers has felt himself to be under excessive pressure. He has described his condition as a feeling of extreme depression which he cannot shake off. Mr. Carl Crackers was admitted to Serenity Acres Psychiatric Hospital, owned and operated by a non-profit organization. The hospital has been granted a charter and is duly licensed as a psychiatric hospital. The staff is comparable to that of an average 200-bed psychiatric institution.

Dr. Sigmund, the chief psychiatrist, has diagnosed Mr. Crackers' condition as schizophrenia-paranoid type with recurrent depression. Mr. Crackers is in contact with reality, and oriented to time, place, and people. However, periodically, he tells the nurses he hears voices telling him to save the world from evil. When talking about these voices, Mr. Crackers begins to get agitated and restless, pacing the floor in his room. Dr. Sigmund has ordered a tranquilizer, 10 mgm. valium taken orally, to be given to Mr. Crackers immediately and then every four hours for two days. Sara Gampie, R.N., takes the medication to Mr. Carl Crackers. Mr. Crackers refuses to take the medication, stating Sara Gampie is trying to poison him. Sara Gampie informs Dr. Sigmund of the situation. Dr. Sigmund tells her the patient must get the medication and any route, oral or intramuscular, is permissible. Dr. Sigmund also tells Sara Gampie that Mr. Crackers might get violent unless he is sedated.

Sara Gampie attempts to give the medication orally again. Mr. Crackers continues to adamantly refuse medication.

What action, if any, should the nurse take in this situation?
What, if any, legal risks are involved?

Answer

There is often a presumption by health professionals that an individual in a psychiatric setting is mentally incompetent *ipso facto*, that is, by that very fact. This is not a valid presumption. In fact, the opposite is true. There is a presumption at law that everyone is presumed to be mentally competent and sane unless there is sufficient evidence to the contrary. There are two methods of commitment to an institution, voluntary and involuntary. If a patient voluntarily enters a treatment center or setting, he can voluntarily leave also. It also follows that such an individual has not given up any of his rights by voluntarily submitting himself for cure. Therefore, such a patient who refuses a medication or a particular treatment is entitled under the law to make that decision and it should be respected. It would follow, therefore, that anyone giving a medication or treatment to a patient clearly in contravention of his stated wishes could be liable for assault and battery.

The patient who is involuntarily committed presents a more difficult problem in trying to ascertain the appropriate legal action to be taken.

Most states have commitment laws. These laws or statutes have criteria to establish that an individual needs medical or psychiatric treatment in a confined setting. In general, the criteria requires that the individual to be confined must be mentally ill and a danger to himself or to members of society.

It is generally necessary that a patient be adjudicated mentally incompetent, that is, that a proper judicial forum implementing all the procedures of due process be convened and give a fair hearing to the issue of establishing the competency or incompetency of the patient.

Mental incompetency is not a medical fact; it is a legal fact based on the medical evidence. Therefore, if a patient is adjudicated mentally incompetent in an appropriate forum, the next question would be who would then be appointed to act as legal guardian for the patient, to make decisions for his general welfare. In some states, a committee is appointed, or a relative, or even the administrator of the particular health care setting makes this decision. The permission for giving medication or treatment to the patient would then rest with those parties. (And any medication or treatment given to the patient adjudicated mentally incompetent without the court-appointed committee's or relative's permission could raise the issue of an assault and battery on the patient.)

There is also the consideration of the patient injuring himself or others. The law would expect the health care practitioners to reasonably protect the patient. It would also expect the hospital as an entity to protect the other patients under its care from potential injury by Mr. Crackers. But any unauthorized treatment of a patient must clearly meet the criteria that the treatment was given to protect the patient or other individuals from harm. Anyone giving such treatment must be prepared to substantiate with facts and evidence that the treatment was given in the best interest of the patient. Merely making the statement is not factual evidence. The activity of the patient and the reasons which necessitated any treatment without proper consent should be well documented and corroborated. The least restrictive method for the patient's safety and the safety of others should be employed.

VIGNETTE 3

RESTRAINTS

Sarah Sack, R.N., is the only registered nurse on a geriatric ward of 35 patients. Every evening for two weeks a particular situation arises with two elderly patients. Mrs. Jennie Gentel, a 72-year-old female, accuses Mrs. Zsa Rudie, an 80-year-old female, of taking her brush and comb. Mrs. Jennie Gentel and Mrs. Zsa Rudie start shouting at each other over this incident and verbally abusing each other. Occasionally, the two patients will get combative and strike each other. In the confusion that results from these encounters, other patients sometimes have been struck inadvertantly by Mrs. Jennie Gentel or Mrs. Zsa Rudie. Sarah Sack has requested Mrs. Jennie Gentel's and Mrs. Zsa Rudie's physician, Dr. Herman Helpful, to write an order for restraints as needed when such occasions arise. Dr. Helpful has consistently refused to write restraining orders because the patients are always quiet when the doctor sees them during the day. The evening supervisor, Clara Bartmelte, R.N., had told Sarah Sack to restrain these patients when she believes it is necessary and the evening supervisor will support her if there is any problem.

Should Sarah Sack, R.N., restrain the patients if she believes it necessary?

Would there be any liability if Sarah Sack, R.N., restrained the patients under the above circumstances?

Would there be any liability if Sarah Sack, R.N., did not restrain the patients under the above circumstances?

Answer

If a patient becomes disturbed or combative, the attending physician should be notified immediately. Restraints should only be used in an emergency to protect the patient or protect other patients from being injured by a combative patient. Restraits generally require a doctor's order. The order for restraint should include the type of restraint to be used and the reason for the restraint. At the same time a nurse must realize she can also be negligent on the basis of *misfeasance* (failing to act when there was a duty to protect the patient).

The freedom from unlawful restraint is an individual freedom protected by law. Unless authorized by law or voluntarily consented to, restraint of any degree constitutes a false imprisonment and is a tort for which one may seek legal redress. Restraints are not to be imposed lightly. To put this in proper perspective, one should realize that the worst punishment society imposes, with the exception of death, is restraint of one's liberty, namely incarceration. Restraint is a form of incarceration. It is not the first step to be taken in control of a patient's behavior, but it should be a last resort after other reasonable means of control have not been satisfactory. It should not be used for administrative or personnel convenience to the detriment of the patient's freedom of movement.

Restraint is used in various degrees in health practice. The mere words, "don't move," pending injection or treatment, as well as the mechanical restraint of a patient ready to be anesthetized are restraints on a patient's freedom. These are reasonable restraints and are not actionable because the patient consents to it either by implied or expressed consent. It is a rather general practice to restrain psychiatric, elderly, sedated and pediatric patients depending on circumstances. However, this should not be done thoughtlessly and each case should be evaluated for need before imposing restraints. The primary purpose for using restraints should be to protect the patient and not to reduce hospital personnel shortage problems or to suit nurses' convenience.

Not only is the decision to use restraints an important one, but the decision to continue restraints is equally important. There is always the danger that the restraints themselves, if not applied properly and checked frequently, may constrict and traumatize the patient. There are situations where restraints have served only to increase a patient's agitation, rather than to alleviate the agitation. Obviously, such a situation is not conducive to furthering quality care; alternative solutions should be sought. Generally, a patient's consent should be obtained when applying necessary restraints. A doctor's order should be obtained when restraints are necessary, unless it is an emergency situation, or unless the patient would injure himself or others if not restrained. Another important consideration is that the restraints are applied primarily for the patient's safety and not for the hospital or nurse's convenience. It is good procedure to consult with another nurse or supervisor regarding the necessity of restraints. If there is concurrence regarding the need for restraints, documentation of the facts and reasons for restraints should be placed in the record and witnessed by a co-worker.

The restraints should be checked frequently to assure they are not too restrictive, are not impairing circulation, or causing pressure sores or other injury. Restraint of the patient should only be maintained for a limited time and for the limited purpose of patient protection. They should be removed at the first opportunity. Even an intravenous solution being given to a patient causes the patient to be restrained, and pressure sores can be caused by taping the patient's arms too tightly. There should be continuous monitoring of the restrained patient. It is a self-evident proposition that a professional person should know when and how to use restraints to adequately protect the disturbed or very young or old patient, with or without prior medical orders, contingent on circumstances. Therefore, a professional will weigh all factors, consider alternatives and then decide to apply or not apply restraints in the best interest of the patient.

VIGNETTE 4

STAFF RELATIONSHIPS, AFFILIATING STUDENTS

Betsy Bump, R.N., is the charge nurse on a surgical unit with 35 patients. This unit has a variety of surgical patients in various stages of post-operative activity. There are generally three to four post-operative gastrectomy, cholecystectomy and colostomy patients. There are also some acutely ill nephrectomy patients and patients receiving hemo-dialysis. Healing Arts Hospital has an affiliation agreement with Clara Barton Community College. Under the agreement this college sends students to receive clinical experience in certain areas. The surgical unit described above is one of the areas chosen for clinical experience. Approximately five students and a clinical instructor, Ida Smart, R.N., M.S., are assigned to the surgical unit every Tuesday and Thursday from 7:30 A.M until 3:00 P.M. From 3:00 to 3:30 P.M., the students and Ida Smart, the instructor, have a post-conference. Every day after the students leave the units, Betsy Bump finds that there are some procedures not completed for the patients assigned to students from Clara Barton Community College. Betsy Bump has been told by Shirley Semple, R.N., Director of Nursing Service, that as charge nurse, she is completely responsible for all the patients on the surgical unit. She has also been told by Shirley Semple, R.N., the same Director of Nursing Services, that Ida Smart, R.N., M.S., instructor from Clara Barton Community College, is totally responsible for the nursing students and that Betsy Bump, R.N., is not to interfere with the students.

> Woud Betsy Bump be at any legal risk in this set of circumstances?
> What action, if any, should Betsy Bump take in this situation?

Answer

There is an inherent contradiction in the position education has placed charge nurses in unless clear policies and understanding between nursing service and education are established. It is well established that the nursing service administration is responsible for quality nursing care. It, therefore, follows that if the student nurse is involved in patient care, and the nursing service administration is responsible for quality nursing care, then nursing service administration must know what kind of care is being given by the student nurses from affiliating schools. It also follows that a nurse who is a charge nurse or a director of nurses who knows, or should know, that incompetent care is being given must take appropriate measures to correct that incompetency. There is a legal duty owed to every patient placed under the nurse's care and jurisdiction. That legal duty to the patient is not displaced by the school of nursing, its instructor or its students. It is true the affiliating instructor is responsible for the students under her charge.

Where there is evidence that the student and/or instructor are not completing the assigned tasks and that the patient may be subjected to possible harm, it is legally incumbent on the nursing service person to take appropriate action. Appropriate action would begin by consulting with the clinical instructor directly. The problem should be attempted to be resolved at this first level. If the nursing service person does not act to protect the patient from being placed at risk, and the patient is injured, it is possible that the nursing service person could be personally liable under the doctrine of foreseeability. That is to say, if the acts of the nursing student or instructor were such that it was reasonable to expect such continued acts could result in harm that reasonable persons could foresee, liability would be justified. For example, a student who has made several medications errors or failed to monitor intravenous fluids may need to be supervised closely. A charge nurse knowing of the student's propensity for error in patient care is not only justified in bringing this to the attention of the instructor, but would be derelict in her professional duty if she did not take action. The conference between the head nurse and instructor should be documented with specific facts, including discussion and action proposed to resolve the problem.

If, after meeting and mutually discussing the situation, the charge nurse and clinical instructor cannot resolve the situation or meet an impasse, then the problem should move to the next level of administration. This might involve the Director of Nursing Service and the Chairman of the Department of Nursing getting involved. The matter should be resolved in the formulation of new policies for the hospital and the college or both institutions. There is no definitive rule of law that students are or are not employees of the college or the hospital. Although the clinical instructor is an employee of the college, it is conceivable that the instructor could in certain circumstances be construed as an "employee" of the hospital. This would increase the possibility of the hospital being held liable for a student and/or clinical instructor's negligent acts.

VIGNETTE 5

COUNTERSIGNING

Nancy Nicer, R.N., has been working at Healing Arts Hospital, Incorporated, for five years. She has worked the evening three-to-eleven shift and the night twelve-to-eight shift. During her work years, she has taken information from various shift personnel and charted the information on the appropriate patient's chart. This has been common practice in the institution. For example, a nursing assistant would test diabetic urine specimens for sugar. The nursing assistant would tell the results to Nancy Nicer, R.N., and Nancy would chart the results.

A new policy is being introduced at the Healing Arts Hospital. The registered nurses are to be required to countersign all entries in the patient's charts and all medications given by nursing staff, including licensed practical nurses and student nurses. The student nurses' notes and medications are also to be countersigned by the clinical instructor.

What, if any, are the legal implications for Nancy Nicer, R.N., if she follows the new policy?
What, if any, are the legal implications for the clinical instructor if she follows the new policy?

Answer

There is a trend to have more persons involved in countersigning various documents used in health care delivery. Before implementing this particular procedure, a health center should review the purpose of countersigning and see if, indeed, that is their objective. Countersigning serves no useful purpose in many instances and could place individuals at legal risk if they are attesting to the authenticity of a statement of a patient or a treatment performed on a patient to which they have never been a party or a first-person observer. The authors are aware that some federal legislation such as medicare may require countersigning by certain health professionals. This, however, should not become a blanket policy in an institution. In fact, if the mandate does not make sense, it should be questioned, government policy or any other policy. Physicians often countersign orders, history and physicals. It is done with the intention of attesting to having given the order previously or of confirming the history and physical examination. This type of countersigning then serves to place the physician in the position of authorizing and/or concurring on that to which he has placed his signature.

This is not the case in some hospitals, where countersigning of nursing students' notes by the college instructor is required according to hospital policy. The stated purpose of this policy is that the hospital requires it. Sometimes the "veiled purpose" is to "force" the instructor to supervise the students more closely. Instead of having a meeting of nursing service and education to discuss supervision of students and develop a mutual solution, a policy such as countersigning is implemented to do indirectly what was not being done directly. This or anything comparable is not the purpose of countersigning. Nurses' aides or assistants often perform certain patient tasks but are not permitted to chart the results of their findings. Instead, the aides convey the results to a nurse, who charts what has been told to her. The nurse often has no personal knowledge of what she is writing. Often she has not seen the patient or the test result and yet she is attesting to the authenticity of events to which she has not been a party.

Anyone who signs a document is presumed to have read the document, and if one places his signature under treatments, medications and notes, it is presumed that the signer has personal knowledge of the information or performed the particular procedure. Therefore, it is incumbent on anyone who purports to give information on a medical record to know the information is accurate. If the handling of the record is for review and medical audit, then the signer should make that clear to the reader. Handlers of medical records often construe the format of the medical record as sacrosanct and hesitate to add anything to a particular form when even if the allotted space provides only room for a checkmark.

The authors are not advocating disregard of form but want to emphasize the need for clarification regardless of format. If it is necessary to add a sentence or even a page to clarify the facts and to protect yourself legally, then do so. Brevity is a commendable attribute. But the essence of effective documentation is the presentation of all the facts. And essential factual information should never be sacrificed in the interest of brevity.

Therefore, if your signature appears on the record in a capacity other than having personal knowledge of the particular events, explain the capacity clearly so in the event of litigation, your position is not misconstrued. Remember that to countersign by definition (Black's *Law Dictionary*) is "to place one's signature to a writing already signed by another to attest to the authenticity of that writing." If your reason for countersigning is not comparable with the definition, it would be judicious to analyze and review your purpose before committing yourself to possible legal risk.

VIGNETTE 6

INFORMED CONSENT

Mrs. Dolly Dimple is a 35-year-old female admitted to Healing Arts Hospital for an elective hysterectomy operation. Mrs. Dimple has signed a routine consent form as required by hospital policy. This was done in the admitting office and witnessed by the admissions clerk. Dolly Dimple has had routine blood drawn and a chest X-ray and has been admitted to the gynecological section of Healing Arts Hospital. Sarah Sack, R.N., has been assigned to prepare Mrs. Dimple for elective surgery. During the course of preparing Mrs. Dimple for surgery, Sarah Sack talks to Mrs. Dolly Dimple about health care in general. Mrs. Dimple states to Sarah Sack, R.N., "My doctor hasn't discussed this surgery with me, but I guess he will before he operates, won't he?" Sarah Sack asks Mrs. Dimple if she signed a consent form to the operation and Mrs. Dimple states, "I signed some kind of consent form when I came in, but I thought that was for hospital tests."

> What, if any, obligation does Sarah Sack, R.N., have toward Mrs. Dolly Dimple?
> Would Sarah Sack, R.N., be liable if Mrs. Smith was operated on under the above circumstances?

Answer

Sarah Sack has several obligations. There is an obligation to the patient, the physician and the hospital. When it becomes evident that the patient, in this case Dolly Dimple, has either not been fully informed of the type of surgery for which she has been admitted or does not understand the implications of the surgery, the patient's physician should be immediately notified. The nurse should document the situation and the fact that the physician was notified. The nurse has an obligation to inform the patient's physician of the patient's statements, so that corrective measures may be taken by the doctor.

The hospital has no direct obligation to inform the patient of the surgical procedure to be done. In fact, it cannot do so since only the surgeon knows what techniques and specific operation will be utilized for the specific patient. But since the hospital could be held as a party-defendant by the patient alleging no consent was given, the nurse should take all reasonable measures to protect the hospital.

The nurse should protect herself, also, because the patient could include the nurse as a party-defendant. The patient has put the nurse on notice that she is uninformed regarding her imminent surgery. The nurse should inform the physician, her immediate supervisor, and any other appropriate parties of the situation. Otherwise the nurse could be held liable if surgery were performed without the patient's consent.

VIGNETTE 7

INFORMED CONSENT SITUATION

Sara Gampie is a staff nurse on the oncology unit at Healing Arts Hospital. She has been caring for Mrs. Molly Moxie, an elderly 72-year-old female patient. Mrs. Moxie has been having trouble breathing for several days. It is getting progressively worse. Dr. Teachem thinks Mrs. Moxie's thoracic cavity has fluid as a result of her lung cancer. Dr. Teachem wants to do a thoracentesis on Mrs. Moxie. He has written the order, "Prepare patient for thoracentesis, stat."

Dr. Teachem also tells Sara Gampie to get a consent form signed by Mrs. Moxie, that she consents to the procedure for a thoracentesis. As Sara Gampie begins to explain the procedure to Mrs. Moxie, Mrs. Moxie asks that her daughter be contacted to give permission before the procedure begins. Sara Gampie has tried several times to contact Mrs. Moxie's daughter but is unable to reach her. Dr. Teachem states he has to go ahead with the procedure or the patient will go into heart failure.

> What, if anything, should Sara Gampie do?
> Can Dr. Teachem proceed with the thoracentesis? If so, under what circumstances?
> What, if any, legal liabilities could be involved?

Answer

There is nothing in the situation to indicate Mrs. Moxie is not competent and capable to consenting to the procedure herself. The patient may consent or withhold consent for medical treatment. The fact that Mrs. Moxie wants her daughter contacted should be respected. The daughter should be notified as requested. Mrs. Moxie may wish to consult with her daughter before submitting to the thoracentesis procedure. However, the daughter's consent cannot be substituted for Mrs. Moxie's consent. The fact that Mrs. Moxie is seventy-two years of age has no bearing on her right to make decisions regarding her own body. Unless there is some evidence of incompetency or inability, only Mrs. Moxie can give an informed consent for the procedure.

Sara Gampie should be reasonably assured that Dr. Teachem has explained the procedure and that Mrs. Moxie understands the situation and have Mrs. Moxie sign the consent form.

Dr. Teachem could proceed with the thoracentesis only if Mrs. Moxie gave an informed consent as outlined above. It would be wise and good business for the daughter to be incorporated into the consent procedure since the patient specifically requested this, but the daughter cannot authorize the procedure where the patient is capable of consenting. It is not an emergency at this point and Dr. Teachem could not proceed under the Emergency Rule as explained in the consent section of this book. He must have the patient's valid consent.

If the above was not done in accord with general practice in procurring consents and the patient could establish she did not give a valid consent, the physician, nurse and hospital might be sued and found liable for assault and battery.

Addendum to Answer 6 and 7

The first amendment guarantees the integrity of one's body. Any touching of an individual's body without appropriate authority or the individual's consent could be construed as an assault and battery. The courts recognize assault and battery as giving rise to a criminal action for which the law gives a remedy in money damages.

Judge Cardozo, a Supreme Court Justice and eminent legal scholar, clearly held that every competent adult had the right to self-determination regarding his body. He further stated any surgeon who performs surgery without the patient's consent commits an assault. This was in 1914 before the fashionable term, "informed consent." The case was *Schloendorf v. Society of New York Hospital*, 211 N.Y. 125 (1914).

It is generally accepted that there is an implicit consent to certain routine procedures by the very fact a patient voluntarily seeks admission to a health care center and requests treatment. However, there is general consensus that a specific consent is required for non-routine procedures.

In general, consent forms show voluntary submission to procedure, not necessarily understanding of procedures.

The hospital and its employees, as well as the doctor, can be held liable for performing a treatment or procedure without the patient's consent. The courts apply the doctrine of corporate liability, respondeat superior or other appropriate law and where it can be ascertained that the hospital, as in this case, knew or should have known there was no bona fide informed consent by the patient and did not correct the situation but permitted uninformed surgery, the nurse, physician and hospital are at legal risk.

Consent to a procedure may be given by anyone who has reached the age of majority in the particular jurisdiction and is not under any legal disability. The law uses the term, *sui juris*, "of his right, possessing full civil rights."

Some criteria should be met by the nurse to assure that proper consent is obtained. The patient must be conscious and able to comprehend the document that is being signed. There should be a reasonable belief on the part of the nurse that the patient has been informed regarding the nature and purpose of the procedure and the possible risks related to it. The patient should be able to read, write and understand the language being used for communication. The patient should be consenting to the procedure freely, voluntarily, and without any coercion (*sua sponte*, "of his own will").

VIGNETTE 8

ILLEGIBLE ORDERS

Nancy Nicer, R.N., has been working at Healing Arts Hospital Incorporated for six months. She has been placed in charge of the medical floor. Her responsibilities include the coronary care unit. Dr. Willis is the private physician for three of the 10 patients in the coronary care unit. Dr. Willis consistently writes medication orders that are illegible and difficult to read. The nurses on the unit have consistently asked Dr. Willis to either write more legibly or tell a nurse on the floor what the written order says before leaving the floor. Dr. Willis replies by saying he has practiced medicine in this hospital for 20 years and never had a problem and that Nancy Nicer and the other nurses could just learn to read his writing.

What, if any, legal risk is involved in this situation?
What, if any, action should be taken by Nancy Nicer and the nurses?

Answer

The illegible medication order is a potentially litigious situation. Every doctor's order must be readable, and in the case of a medication, the amount and route of administration must be clearly indicated. If a doctor consistently leaves illegible orders, this should be brought to the particular physician's attention, including the effects of such illegibility on daily functions—for example, the amount of time lost spent in trying to read and decipher the order, time wasted in trying to contact the writer as well as the danger of giving wrong medications, or the wrong amount. Often, the problem is resolved when the physician and nurse discuss the issue as professional colleagues working for the patient's best interest. If the physician persists in writing illegible orders or ignores or berates the nurse, then the appropriate channels must be followed. The medical director in an institution can be an excellent resource person in bringing about mutually acceptable solutions for inter-professional problems.

The nurse cannot execute an order she cannot read. This is basic. The nurse would be considered negligent if she were to perform a function or give a medication on the basis that she thought that is what the illegible order stated and she was wrong. She would be liable for any injuries resulting to the patient under these circumstances. The literature is full of examples where nurses have taken a chance and attempted to follow illegible orders. The reasonably-prudent-man doctrine would be most applicable, because no reasonably prudent nurse would act on an illegible order and permit herself to be placed in such obvious legal jeopardy.

VIGNETTE 9

LEAVING AGAINST MEDICAL ADVICE

Clara Bartonette is the supervisor on evening duty, 3:30 P.M. to 12 midnight at Healing Arts Hospital, Incorporated. The emergency room is always a busy unit, especially on the weekends. On this particular Saturday, at 11:00 P.M., Clara Bartonette, R.N., receives a call from Adela Nursey, R.N., head nurse in the Shock-Trauma-Emergency Unit. Adela Nursey relays the following to Clara Bartonette, supervisor: A patient, Fannie Fussie, 64 years old, came to the Emergency Room at 8:00 P.M. in a city ambulance. Mrs. Fussie slipped and fell on her kitchen floor. She was able to reach a telephone and call for help. Mrs. Fussie has been X-rayed and the X-ray shows a linear fracture to her left femur. The area is swollen and tender to touch.

Mrs. Fussie has been lying on the stretcher in the hallway for two hours because the emergency room was full and there were no beds to put Mrs. Fussie into when she came from x-ray. Mrs. Fussie is very upset at the lack of attention and apparent and apparent lack of concern on the part of the hospital staff. She wishes to leave the hospital. She has told the head nurse she wants to leave immediately. The doctor assigned to the emergency room, Dr. Irvin, and the head nurse, Adela Nursey, have explained to Mrs. Fussie that she has a fractured femur and to leave without being treated and having a cast applied could lead to serious complications. Dr. Irvin also informed the patient that the hospital would not be responsible. He asks Mrs. Fussie to sign the hospital form indicating she has been properly advised of her condition, has refused treatment, and is leaving against medical advice. Mrs. Fussie refuses to sign anything without a lawyer being present. She insists she wants to leave the hospital and is becoming progressively upset by the entire situation.

Adela Nursey asked Clara Bartonette to advise her what action to take in this situation.

> What, if any, legal risks are involved for Dr. Irvin, Clara Bartonette, and Adela Nursey in this situation?
> Would there be any liability for Healing Arts Hospital, Incorporated, under these circumstances.

Answer

There is a general principle in law that every adult who is mentally competent has the legal right to accept or reject any medical treatments. The attending physician or hospital representative should explain to the patient the medical risk involved in leaving the emergency room against medical advice. If, after such explanation, the patient persists in wishing to leave, a document or form "Against Medical Advice" should be signed by the patient and witnessed. If the patient refuses to sign such a document, a clear recitation of all events that took place in the emergency room should be written on the patient's record and a co-worker or colleague who witnessed the events should sign the record as well as the supervisor.

There are times in the hospital setting when patients cannot get immediate attention because of other priorities. For example, a coronary patient may get attention over a patient with abdominal pain. Or a shot-wound patient may take priority over a patient with a fracture. Assuming that the emergency room staff were performing their duties as well as could be expected, and assuming that, although the two-hour delay was a long time, it could not have been shortened under the circumstances, there would be no liability for any of the parties in this situation.

Mrs. Fussie has had the risks of her leaving against medical advice explained to her. She is a competent adult and if she elects to leave the hospital after all reasonable attempts have been made to explain the situation, she does so at her own risk. The law clearly permits an individual to make decisions which are not in their own best health interests. Health care practitioners may not agree with the individual patient's decisions regarding his health care but they may not interfere with the exercise of that decision.

VIGNETTE 10

EMPLOYEE RELATIONSHIPS

Sara Gampie, R.N., is the head nurse on a 25-bed surgical unit at Healing Arts Hospital, Incorporated. One of her job functions is to prepare the work schedules for all three shifts—day, evening and night. The schedules are prepared and posted at least two months in advance. Sara Gampie scheduled herself to work evenings on the first weekend in May. Daisy Dilatory, a nursing technician, was also scheduled to work evenings that particular weekend. Daisy Dilatory did not appear for work on the weekend as scheduled, nor did she call or send any messages to Sara Gampie regarding her absence. This type of situation has happened before with Daisy. Sara Gampie was unable to get a substitute for Daisy and had to care for the entire unit by herself as a result of Daisy's unexpected absence.

Sara Gampie is concerned about caring for all 25 patients by herself. She realizes she will be unable to give adequate care to all the patients. Sara notifies the evening supervisor, Clara Bartonette, R.N., of the situation and her concern. Clara Bartonette said she is unable to send any other staff, because two nurses from Intensive Care called in sick, and the entire hospital is short-staffed. Clara tells Sara Gampie to do the best she can and if there is any change in staff, she will send help.

On Monday evening Daisy comes to work on the unit. Sara Gampie asks Daisy for an explanation of the failure to come to work as scheduled and the failure to notify anyone of the absence so appropriate measures could be taken.

Daisy Dilatory states she got mixed up and thought she was off that particular weekend.

What, if anything, should Sara Gampie do regarding this situation?

Answer

Because the hospital has a duty to each and every patient admitted for care to its premises, it has an obligation to implement standards to assure quality care will be maintained. Implicit in this obligation is the right to develop and maintain policies, procedures, rules and regulations which give information and guidance to employees who work in the institution. The employee has certain rights also. He has a right to know the policies of the hospital and what is expected of him as an employee. He also has a right to know what, if anything, will happen if he fails to meet those expectations set out in his job description, or in the policies and procedures of the hospital.

The employee who consistently fails to appear for work without notifying his superior or giving an explanation for this unacceptable behavior is subject to disciplinary action. The disciplinary action should be according to the policy of the hospital. Any procedural steps or protocol spelled out in the policy should be followed conscientiously. The nurse should use clear and concise language in documenting what has taken place. The conference or discussion with the employee should be included. If a future course of action has been decided between the nurse and the technician, that also should be included.

Either the employee should have the opportunity to read the memorandum made by the nurse and sign it, or a copy of the memorandum should be given to the employee or both, depending on hospital procedure.

The memorandum should state facts and what the nurse perceived through her senses to be a fact. Judgmental terms and conclusions should be scrupulously avoided.

The employee should have the opportunity to review the document prepared by Sara Gampie. Daisy Dilatory should be requested to sign the document evidencing the fact that she has been notified of the particular information. If employee Daisy Dilatory refuses to sign the document, this should be noted. A copy of the document should be sent to the appropriate parties, such as the Director of Nurses and Personnel Director.

VIGNETTE 11

INADEQUATE CARE AND INCOMPETENT STAFF

Adela Nursey, R.N., is the head nurse for the Healing Arts Hospital emergency room. Sara Slash, R.N., is a staff nurse in the emergency room. Sara has been working in the emergency room for the past six months. Adela Nursey has been head nurse for two years. For the past six months, Sara Slash has been observing the medical care given by Dr. Bimbo in the emergency room. Sara believes the care is inadequate and incompetent. She bases her belief on the fact that she has observed Dr. Bimbo contaminating equipment and continuing to use it. Dr. Bimbo often does not follow hospital policy, will not write the verbal orders he has given during an emergency, following the emergency. There were two occasions when he corrected the nurses on duty in front of patients.

On a particular Friday night, Dr. Bimbo was called to the emergency room for an accident case. The patient was hemorrhaging and going into shock. Dr. Bimbo arrived 20 minutes after being called. He was irate and began by telling the nurses he should have been called sooner. The patient was in profound shock, bleeding but conscious, and could hear the hostile doctor—nurse interchange. These and similar incidents have been occurring with other staff nurses and Dr. Bimbo, but Sara Slash seems to be the only nurse offended by these incidents. Sara Slash has written a memo to Clara Bartonette, supervisor, outlining the incidents which she feels indicate incompetent patient care being practiced by Dr. Bimbo in the Emergency Room.

> What, if anything, should be the action taken by Clara Bartonette, supervisor, R.N., in this set of circumstances?
> What, if any, further action should be taken by Sara Slash, R.N.?
> What, if any, legal implications or legal risks are involved?

Answer

This is a relatively common complaint among nurses. It is a dilemma that often seems to have no resolution, because factual documentation of the alleged incidents are often not made.

The first action to be taken by Clara Bartonette is to get all the facts. This means several things. Hearsay information is not sufficient.

If possible, Clara Bartonette should arrange to observe the actions of Dr. Bimbo herself. If this is not feasible, she should try to get corroboration of the events that Sara Slash has related in her memo.

This is a potentially dangerous situation. There is legal risk for each individual in this set of facts. Everyone working in Healing Arts Hospital has the obligation to give proper care to the patients under his care. This includes protecting the patient from any harm. Meeting the standard of care due a patient includes taking affirmative action in certain circumstances. This is an example of those certain circumstances. Clara Bartonette has been put on notice that the patients are receiving less than adequate care. It is legally incumbent upon her to assess the situation and move to correct any situations that are potentially dangerous for the patient. Clara Bartonette may think it appropriate to begin with Dr. Bimbo and Sara Slash to work towards a solution. She may think it more appropriate to discuss the situation with the administration. The point is that she must take affirmative action to protect the patients. In the event of injury to a patient because of Dr. Bimbo's activities, Clara Bartonette might be deemed negligent for her inaction.

Sara Slash has to be careful to be very objective and factual in her presentation of charges against Dr. Bimbo. Dr. Bimbo has a license to practice medicine. He has privileges at Healing Arts Hospital, and he is therefore presumed to be practicing appropriately. This does not mean Sara Slash should not pursue the situation, only that she should be aware of this presumption.

If Sara Slash has been observing inadequate and incompetent care by Dr. Bimbo, Sara Slash has a professional obligation and duty to attempt to rectify the situation. The facts set out a situation where patients could be seriously injured in the emergency room. Sara Slash has acted appropriately by notifying the supervisor in writing of what is happening in the emergency room. Sara Slash would be wise to document any and all observed incidents. She should get corroborating witnesses to document these incidents.

In summary, the nursing staff should have corroboration and documentation of the alleged incidents of incompetent and harmful care. The appropriate channels, or chain of command, or hospital policy should be followed to notify the administration so that remedial action, if needed, can be instituted.

The nursing staff should demonstrate that their actions were in the patient's best interests. Their actions were those that similar professionals would take in such circumstances. They had no vested in-

Corroboration: confirmation

terest, were not involved in a vendetta. They were acting without bias or prejudice. They were motivated by professional concern for proper patient care.

Finally, as employees of the hospital, they are protecting the hospital's interests by notifying administration of potentially litiguous situations in the emergency room or other areas. This is a legal and ethical responsibility of any professional person.

VIGNETTE 12

PRIVACY CASE

Dolly Dimple, R.N., is a staff nurse at Healing Arts Hospital working in the Coronary Care Unit for two years. Recently, a new nurse, Tottie Talker, has been sent to the unit for orientation to prepare her to work on the 3 to 11 shift in the Coronary Care Unit. Ms. Dimple notices Tottie Talker talks to all the patients, asking them many questions of a personal nature not related to their care. This is a 10-bed unit.

One day, Dolly Dimple and Tottie Talker were assigned to the same lunch period. While on the way to the cafeteria, the two nurses were on the elevator and Tottie Talker began to discuss Mrs. Masie West. Tottie Talker said Mrs. West told her she had been living with a prominent surgeon who was on the staff and had an illegitimate child by him. Tottie Talker continued, non-stop, relating incidents about Mrs. West.

Dolly Dimple was concerned about Tottie Talker's monologue regarding Mrs. West. There were other people on the elevator. Tottie seemed completely unaware of the other parties on the elevator.

What, if any, legal implications are involved in this set of circumstances?

Answer

Discussing patient's cases on elevators, in cafeterias, or other public areas is a breach of the fiduciary trust and right to confidentiality to which patients are entitled as part of the "due care" owed by the institution. It can also be an invasion of privacy. This right to privacy was interpreted by the U.S. Supreme Court to exist for every citizen as part of the Constitutional rights and is, therefore, an inherent right. The First Amendment which gives freedom of speech and religion has been interpreted as protecting the citizen's right to privacy.

It is unethical and unprofessional conduct to discuss anything of a private or personal nature concerning the patient. This is one of the most abused areas in patient relations. In the past, there was segregation in most hospitals for hospital employees and visitors and this physical separation prevented visitors overhearing employees' conversations. Today, most hospitals share all facilities and more contact between hospital personnel and visitors result. If hospital personnel are not cognizant of their professional responsibility not to reveal any information about the patient, they should know that the discussions that take place between the patient and the hospital personnel are considered confidential communications. Any access to the patient's records or other data would come under the same classification.

The patient, as in this case, has the right to be protected from any disclosure of information that would embarrass, stigmatize, or cause her to be held in less esteem.

This is not the same as privileged communication. Privileged communication has special protection under the law. It has traditionally been recognized to exist between an attorney and client, clergyman and church member, psychiatrist and patient. Where communication is privileged, the confidence entrusted in the course of the professional capacity cannot be revealed and has special immunities.

All professional associations are governed by a code of ethics that addresses itself to the issue of not repeating or communicating any information relating to the patient without appropriate or justifiable reasons.

This is obviously a necessary requirement so patients may feel free to discuss their problems, their illnesses and other personal matters, in the full assurance that nothing will be repeated. The law considers the unnecessary disclosure of confidential information improper. To discuss the patient's confidential information with a third party is a breach of confidence. It is an unlawful disclosure for which the patient may have a cause of action against the party revealing such information.

VIGNETTE 13

RESUSCITATION

Amy Artful, R.N., is the staff nurse in the Coronary Care Unit of Healing Arts Hospital. The unit has a capacity of 10 patients and is usually filled to capacity.

Amy Artful was working the 12:00 midnight to 8:00 A.M. shift on a particular weekend. About two'clock in the morning, an elderly 78-year-old male, Samuel Pepper, is admitted in congestive heart failure. Dr. Greg Heartburn, Mr. Pepper's private physician, is called and he arrives at the Coronary Care Unit shortly after Mr. Pepper.

Dr. Heartburn writes routine orders for Mr. Pepper, including intravenous fluid and medication for pain. Dr. Heartburn then says to nurse Amy Artful, "If Mr. Pepper goes into cardiac arrest, or stops breathing, do not resuscitate him, but I'm not going to put that order in writing."

Around 5 A.M. Mr. Pepper begins to fibrillate. His heart and respirations cease and Mr. Pepper begins to get cyanotic.

What, if anything, should Amy Artful do in these circumstances?

What, if any, would be the legal liabilities for action taken by Amy Artful?

Answer

This situation is one which can arise where the physician is concerned about possible litigation. He therefore refuses to put in writing what he is willing to verbally tell a nurse often in the presence of others. The nurse should not be subjected or ever allow herself to be subjected to such ambiguous tactics. It is quite understandable why the physician might act in the manner described, but it does not resolve any problems and creates difficulty for the nurse.

A verbal order is a legal order. The doctor who gives a verbal order to a nurse is giving a valid order. The doctor who gives a verbal order in the presence of witnesses is giving a valid order with corroborating evidence. The fact that the physician refuses to write the order does not change the validity. There may be a question of proof if the doctor later repudiates or denies he never gave such an order. If any litigation results and there are contradictory statements between the doctor and nurse, the issue may come down to credibility, the credibility of the doctor or the nurse.

First, one must understand that the law presumes every individual wants to preserve his life. The law further presumes that the individual wishes to preserve his life through the ordinary means available. The law does not presume the individual would want extraordinary measures to be taken in the preservation of life. There is no clear distinction at law between what is ordinary and what is extraordinary. The extraordinary means of a few decades ago are the ordinary means of today. So such distinctions must take into consideration many factors, psychological, sociological, economical and technological factors, to name a few. For example, the price of a kidney dialysis machine for an indigent patient might be considered extraordinary, whereas to a Rockefeller or J. Paul Getty, the cost would be considered in the realm of ordinary. Others classify ordinary means on a philosophical basis, that is, anything other than the natural means to resuscitate would be extraordinary. Therefore, any type of machinery would by the narrow interpretation of this definition be construed to be extraordinary.

If the physician makes such an assessment, he should be willing to write an order to that effect. This is a medical judgment and should not be made by the nurse. What should the nurse do if the doctor refuses to write the order? The nurse must follow hospital policy or protocol or procedure in lieu of written direction by the physician. But it is also incumbent on her to bring this situation to the attention of administration through appropriate channels and with appropriate documentation. This establishes that the nurse is acting as a professional and in the best interest of the patient and hospital.

As generally expected, such actions would follow the nurse's attempt to discuss the problem with the attending physician to work out a solution. But no nurse should be placed in such a dilemma without physicians' orders, policy, and procedures or guidelines to assist her in making the best possible professional judgments.

The resuscitation procedure was never intended to be utilized as a routine procedure for all patients. Its purpose was to revive those who had been victims of sudden, traumatic types of expiration. The purpose was to revive those who could live a meaningful and viable life following such resuscitation. Like any procedure, there should be medical criteria for the implementation of resuscitative efforts and applied on a case by case method.

VIGNETTE 14

DENYING HEROIC MEASURES

Olive Oggle, R.N., is a staff nurse working in the Oncology Unit of Healing Arts Hospital, Incorporated. She has been working on the unit for six months. She has been caring for patients in various stages of cancer. For the past month, Ms. Oggle has been the primary nurse for Lennie Lukas. Mr. Lukas, a 55-year-old male, has been diagnosed as having cancer of the lung, terminal stage. Mr. Lukas' physician has indicated that Mr. Lukas has approximately a month to live.

Olive Oggle, R.N., has worked with Mr. Lukas and his family to help them accept the diagnosis and the inevitability of Mr. Lukas' death. Olive Oggle has a good relationship with both Mr. and Mrs. Lukas. One evening, Mrs. Lukas approaches Olive Oggle, R.N., and tells her that no heroic measures are to be used on Mr. Lukas if his condition worsens. Mrs. Lukas further states that has not discussed this with her husband, but that she knows her husband would not want heroic measures and she forbids it.

What, if any, reaction would be appropriate for Olive Oggle?

Answer

In such an emotionally charged situation, the nurse should listen attentively to the patient's family and their concerns. However, the nurse must remember that a patient who is competent has the right to make the decisions that involve his or her life. The health care delivery system is prone to develop the attitude that a seriously ill patient is somehow under a legal handicap. Because there is this "perception," if there is a medical handicap resulting from sickness, there is a tendency to deny the patient certain rights and to permit the others, that is family or physicians, to substitute their judgment for the patient's judgment. The patient is the only one who can legally make these judgments determining if heroic measures shall be employed.

There have been attempts to anticipate such events by executing a document that has been called a "living will." Thus far, the living will is not legally binding, unless enacted statutorily by the legislatures of the respective states. Several state legislatures have introduced legislation which would permit an individual to declare what he would wish to be done in the event that he becomes terminally ill or irrevocably handicapped. This type of legislation is extremely controversial. There seems to be no basic agreement whether individuals have the right to order that no life-saving mechanisms be utilized for them. Certain religious affiliations believe this is usurping the right of God to determine life and death. Other groups of persons who agree an individual has this right over their body, disagree as to the physician's role or the hospital's role in coming to such decisions. Some believe this too awesome a power to be given to health care providers.

In view of the ambiguity of the situation and the legal risks involved in such situations, the health care center should have clear and definite policy and guidelines to assist the nurse in making professional decisions which relate to the decision of life and death. The resource persons and the persons delegated with the authority to handle such complex situations must be clearly designated and available at all times for assistance.

If an interdisciplinary committee to assist the patient and family is functioning at the respective institutions, the nurse should refer the patient's family to this committee, or other appropriate body. The national trend is to establish such interdisciplinary bodies in health care institutions to assist all citizens in making decisions regarding themselves and their families.

California is the first state which has enacted a statute which gives legal efficacy to the "living will." It has yet to be tested in the court system. But it is the first state to move forward in facing the controversial issues. Oregon has recently followed California's example.

As science and bionics continue to develop technologies and apply them to the health care field, more biomedical, ethical, legal and philosophical issues will evolve. The health care professional will be more involved in making decisions or assisting others to make decisions. Therefore, whatever guidelines and resources needed for these serious and complex decisions should be made available by the health care agency.

VIGNETTE 15

TEACHING HOSPITALS

Healing Arts Hospital, Incorporated, has an affiliation agreement with the schools of medicine and nursing at the nearby university. As part of the agreement, the students from the university are permitted to utilize the clinical facilities for teaching and learning experiences. Judi Jumpi, R.N., is the head nurse in the out-patient department. She is familiar with the affiliation agreement and the hospital policy and the fact that Healing Arts Hospital is considered a teaching hospital. Mrs. Gritty is a 25-year-old female who has been having a whitish vaginal discharge for the past two weeks. She has been a gynecological patient at Healing Arts Hospital utilizing the clinic services from time to time in the Out Patient Department.

Dr. Teachem is the staff physician assigned to teaching rounds and is responsible for three students of medicine. Dr. Teachem asks

Judy Jumpi, R.N., to prepare Mrs. Gritty for a vaginal examination. During the preparation, Dr. Teachem informs Judy Jumpi to have sufficient equipment because each student is to examine Mrs. Gritty by doing a vaginal examination. Mrs. Gritty has not been told that these extra examinations are to be done. Judy Jumpi is concerned about such a procedure. Judy Jumpi is not certain whether Mrs. Gritty must be informed about medical students doing procedures since this is a teaching hospital.

What, if any, legal implications could be involved in this set of circumstances?
What, if any, rights does Mrs. Gritty have in these circumstances?

Answer

There is often a misconception among health care practitioners that a patient who is admitted to a teaching hospital automatically becomes a subject for teaching, learning and practicing procedures. This is not correct. Patients do not waive any rights, constitutional or otherwise, because they are treated in an institution which also educates health care practitioners. It is appropriate for the patient to be informed of who is attending her and under what conditions. All parties working with and for the patient should introduce and identify themselves by name and position to the patient. The patient always has the option of refusing treatment, either the treatment itself or the person purporting to perform the treatment.

The law is clear that admission of nonessential persons during procedures and treatments of a patient constitutes a violation of the right of privacy unless the patient has given consent.

Each of the parties, that is, Dr. Teachem, the three medical students and Judy Jumpi, would be at legal risk for invading the patient's privacy if the unnecessary examinations are for the students' benefit and not for the patient's benefit, and the patient has not been consulted regarding the examinations. The patient also has a right to be examined and treated by licensed, competent and trained health care practitioners. If less qualified persons are to be attending the patient, the patient should be made reasonably aware of this fact. It is, then, up to the patient to accept or reject the particular staff. Each time a patient is subjected to another unnecessary examination, it means added inconvenience. It may mean added discomfort, and possibly the risk of infection. Students are learning and, therefore, presumably not as academically competent and not as skilled at technique as the licensed practitioner. We are living in an era of the consumer's right to know. Certainly, in the area of health care, the patient should be fully informed.

VIGNETTE 16

SPLITTING MEDICATION

Polly Peachpit, R.N., is the primary care nurse for Henry Hassle. Mr. Henry Hassle was admitted to the medical unit of Healing Arts Hospital for abdominal pain of unknown etiology. Dr. Macho is the attending physician for Mr. Hassle. Dr. Macho has written routine admission orders for Mr. Hassle. Among the orders written, Dr. Macho writes an order of Demerol 100 mg. intramuscularly for pain every four hours as needed.

At 4 P.M., as soon as Dr. Macho leaves the floor, Mr. Hassle requests medication for abdominal pain. Polly Peachpit, R.N., administers the 100 mg of Demerol intramuscularly according to the order of Dr. Macho.

At 8:30 P.M., following visiting hours, the nurse's aide informs Polly Peachpit that Henry Hassle has requested some medication for pain. Polly Peachpit decides to verify Mr. Hassle's complaint of pain. Upon asking Mr. Hassle about his complaint of pain, Mr. Hassle responds, "It's not too bad, it's like a toothache." Polly Peachpit decides to give Mr. Hassle 50 mg of Demerol instead of the full dose of 100 mg as ordered by Dr. Macho. She does this based on the rational that (1) Mr. Hassle is not that uncomfortable to warrant a 100 mg of Demerol; (2) she can give Mr. Hassle the other 50 mg later when he becomes uncomfortable again; (3) it is common practice on the floor to split pain medications when the nurse determines the patient is not in severe pain.

Is this a proper method of procedure for Polly Peachpit?
What, if any, are the legal risks involved?

Answer

The immediate questions that arise in this fact situation are: "Is the nurse practicing medicine by splitting medications or reducing the amount of Demerol ordered?" Or, "Is the nurse making a professional judgment in adjusting the amount of medication according to the condition of the patient?"

Traditionally the nurse may not diagnose or prescribe for a patient. This is the prerogative of the doctor and is considered to be a medical act. The nurse who alters the amount of medication ordered by the physician without a specific order could be construed as practicing medicine, an illegal act.

The unlicensed practice of medicine, law, nursing or any other profession or occupation required by the police power of the state to have a license constitutes a criminal offense. Licensure is the process by which an agency of the government grants to persons meeting certain qualifications the right to practice a certain profession or engage in a certain occupation. The police power of the state is the power to enact and enforce laws to protect the health, safety and general welfare of the people of the state. It therefore follows that the process of licensure is an attempt to assure that only qualified persons are in a position to exert an effect on the health, safety and general welfare of the people.

The nurse has a license to practice nursing. She does not have a license to practice medicine. Polly Peachpit was actually practicing medicine without a license. This is an illegal act. It is the physician's prerogative to diagnose and prescribe. When Polly Peachpit administered 50 mg of Demerol in place of the 100 mg of Demerol ordered, she was in fact prescribing. Polly Peachpit has no authority to do this under her nursing license. The physician did not delegate any authority to change his order. Even if the physician were to tell Polly Peachpit, "Use your own judgment," the law would consider this improper. The physician cannot authorize the nurse to practice medicine without a license.

The fact that splitting medications has become common procedure on the unit does not give any authority for this practice.

Orders given by the physician are binding on the nurse. The nurse cannot substitute her judgment or preempt the physician's responsibility to treat the patient. If circumstances have changed substantially from those under which the doctor prescribed certain orders, these facts should be brought to the prescribing physician's attention. The nurse who changes a doctor's order without the knowledge and consent of that doctor could be charged with committing a criminal act, an act in violation of state statutes which determines the practice of medicine.

VIGNETTE 17

CONTRACT

Monte Moneychips is a very rich, elderly patient. He is considered to be a multimillionaire. It is rumored he made his money manufacturing home-made beer and liquor during the prohibition period in the early

1930's. Monte Moneychips has been a patient at Healing Arts Hospital for six months. He was originally admitted for a stroke. Since his original admission, Monte Moneychips has had several small brain hemorrhages. The physical impairment resulting from the brain hemorrhage has in no way impaired Monte's mental acuity. He is clear, lucid, competent and alert.

Greta Greedy, R.N., has been caring for Monte Moneychips as a special duty nurse for the past two months. She is an excellent nurse, very proficient and has special ability in caring for cardio-vascular accident patients. Mr. Moneychips is pleased with the care he has received from Greta Greedy.

One afternoon, Monte Moneychips promises to leave his faithful nurse, Greta Greedy, R.N., a bequest in his will of $50,000 for all her care and considerations. Monte Moneychips said he wanted Greta Greedy to have economic security for the rest of her days. He further said she would be able to retire from the nursing profession.

Several witnesses heard Mr. Moneychips make this statement several days before he died. In reviewing the last will and testament of Mr. Moneychips, attorneys found no reference to the bequest of $50,000 to Greta Greedy, R.N. The executor-attorney, I. M. Sharpie, refuses to honor the promise made by Monte Moneychips in the presence of witnesses.

Greta Greedy, R.N., sues the estate of Monte Moneychips, alleging all the above and demanding the money be paid to her under the law of contracts.

What are Greta Greedy's rights in this situation?

Answer

This is an unenforceable promise. The court would probably find the services performed were voluntary or that she had already been paid for them and no promise to pay more for the services performed is enforceable. She did not change her position relying on the promise. That is, Greta Greedy did not quit her job or retire, relying on Monte's promise. If she had done so, it may have made a difference in the court's mind. But ordinarily where there is simply an empty promise to give a gift to another party, the court cannot enforce the payment of a gift.

As a special duty nurse, Greta Greedy was paid for her particular services. Therefore, Monte Moneychips was under no legal obligation

Bequest: an amount of personal properties

to do anything other than pay her for the nursing services for which she was employed.

The courts would generally rule in favor of the executor of the estate of Monte Moneychips who refused to pay the money under the circumstances.

VIGNETTE 18

DEFECTIVE EQUIPMENT

Sara Gampie, R.N., has been working at Healing Arts Hospital for over 20 years. She was trained at the hospital over 25 years ago when the hospital had a school of nursing. During the time of training, Sara Gampie, R.N., was taught that one of the qualities of a professional nurse is the ability to improvise. Sara Gampie has been "improvising" as necessity indicated all her professional life. There were often times when equipment was not adequate and Sara Gampie always managed on the unit with the equipment given to her by administration.

She has been working in the recovery room for the past few months on the day shift. The suction machine that is being used for Mrs. Daily Doosie, a post-operative laryngectomy, does not seem to be functioning properly. Sara Gampie thinks there isn't sufficient pressure being generated by the machine's motor. By pressing on the tube in two or three places while the motor is running, the suction machine seems to function better.

When giving change of shift report to Fannie Funnie, the staff nurse in the recovery room for the 3-to-11 shift, Sara Gampie explains the condition of the suction machine. Sara tells Fannie Funnie if she presses on the tube in two places, the pressure stays up sufficiently to suction Mrs. Doosie. Sara tells Fannie she could utilize this method if necessary during the evening shift until the defective equipment is fixed in the morning.

What, if any, are the legal risks involved in this situation?

Answer

One important duty of the nurse is to ascertain that the equipment used in procedures and treatments is free from defects. The equipment must be appropriate for the purposes for which it is to be used. There are essentially two elements to be considered for this particular duty. First, reasonably prudent care must be exercised in selecting specific equipment for a specific purpose. Second, reasonably prudent care must be exercised in the maintenance of the equipment.

If the manufacturer's instructions require periodic inspections or other requirements to insure optimum functioning, such instructions should be followed. The nurse may or may not be primarily responsible for such inspections. But the nurse is always responsible for reasonable action in a situation. If the nurse observes that equipment is not functioning properly, the prudent action is to have it corrected by the individual responsible for its functioning at optimum level. The responsibility factor depends on several things, the situation itself, size of the hospital or health center, number of staff available and comparable components. If the nurse is in any way responsible for equipment functioning properly, it is wise to have documentation of the times the equipment is checked and found to be working properly, or if defects are found, that defects are corrected, when and by whom. There can be liability imposed on the nurse and the hospital if equipment, facilities and health systems fail to function properly. This does not mean the health care center must have the latest or the most expensive equipment. But what it does have must be free from defects, operating at optimum capacity and used by personnel who have been trained to use the equipment if special training is necessary.

In the case presented where the nurse has been put on notice by the head nurse that the equipment is "acting funny," the potential for possible injury to the two patients needing suction is clear. Patients with orders to "suction P.R.N." are depending on properly functioning equipment. It is evident that failure to suction a patient properly when body fluids accumulate could result in death for the patient. The law would probably consider this a foreseeable event. The law could also look to see if the nurse acted as reasonably prudent nurses would have acted in the same set of circumstances. That is, the nurse could reasonably foresee that properly functioning equipment would be needed for certain patients. The nurse has a legal duty to see that the equipment used for patient care is in good condiiton. The nurse should contact the appropriate supervisor or personnel to obtain adequite suctioning equipment. A memorandum of the situation might be necessary to substantiate that the nurse acted in a reasonably prudent manner if there is any question of legal risk.

VIGNETTE 19

SUPERVISION

Sara Bartonette, R.N., is the evening supervisor for Healing Arts Hospital, Incorporated. She has been evening supervisor for 15 years. While making rounds one evening, an elderly patient, John Jeppi, 78

years of age, complained to Sara Bartonette of being excessively cold.
Clara Gampie, R.N., is the charge nurse on the floor. Sara Bartonette
goes to Clara Gampie and tells her Mr. Jeppi is complaining of being
cold and to "take care of it and see that Mr. Jeppi is made more comfortable." Clara Gampie is busy talking to Dr. Macho about another
patient on the floor. Clara Gampie asked Dr. Macho to write an order
for a hot water bottle for Mr. Jeppi. Dr. Macho wrote the order as
requested. Thereafter, Clara Gampie tells Fannie Fidget, L.N.P., to
give Mr. Jeppi a hot water bottle for his feet to make him more comfortable. Fannie Fidget applied a hot water bottle shortly afterwards
in accordance with the direction of Clara Gampie.

Mr. Jeppi's feet became blistered within one hour of the application of the hot water bottle. Dr. Macho was called to examine Mr.
Jeppi's feet. Dr. Macho diagnosed the area of blistering on Mr. Jeppi's
feet as first and second degree burns caused by the hot water bottle.
Dr. Macho also said the poor circulation in Mr. Jeppi's feet due to
his age was a factor in the burning.

Who would be held liable in this situation, and why?

Answer

The supervisor has a responsibility for the quality of care given
to the patients under her jurisdiction. She is held to the standard of
care that other supervisors in the same set of circumstances would be
expected to meet. One of the expectations of a supervisor's activity is
that she will make proper surveillance of the care patients receive
from the staff to be certain it is competent, skilled and safe.

In this factual situation, Sara Bartonette, the evening supervisor
has requested that a hot water bottle be given to a patient. This is
not an unusual request. It certainly is within the scope of a registered
nurse or a licensed practical nurse to perform this function.

One of the implied commitments a hospital makes to the staff it
employs is that the hospital will have competent personnel, equipment, and facilities with which the employees can work. Both Sara
Bartonette and Clara Gampie have a right to assume that nursing
service has checked the credentials of the people with whom they are
working. They have a right to presume these same persons are competent, unless put on notice to the contrary. Assuming the equipment
used was not defective, it would seem Fannie Fidget was negligent in
the application of the hot water bottle and caused the injury to John
Jeppi's foot. The fact that Mr. Jeppi was 78 years old and had poor

circulation might be mitigating. But it would more likely be even more damaging. A reasonably prudent nurse should have the nursing judgment to give higher care to an elderly patient with poor circulation. It is common knowledge such patients' skin is more sensitive and susceptible to burning. Assuming all the elements of negligence were established, Fannie Fidget would be liable for the damages incurred by Mr. Jeppi.

Neither Sara Bartonette nor Clara Gampie would be responsible for Fannie Fidget's negligence. The nursing function delegated to Fannie was a proper one and within her expected scope of ability. They had never been put on notice that Fannie was not competent in applying hot water bottles. However, now they have been put on notice. Before Fannie can again apply hot water bottles to patients, several things should be done.

First, there should be an ascertaining of how the injury happened. Was Fannie simply careless? Did Fannie check the temperature of the water? Did she follow the hospital procedure? Once the cause is established, then remedial measures should be taken relative to the cause. It is ncessary that some retraining take place and documentation of that retraining be made before Fannie Fidget can function safely in applying hot water bottles.

No one is responsible for another's negligence unless he contributed to or participated in that negligence. The head nurse or supervisor is not legally responsible for the negligent actions of those supervised unless they in fact contributed to that negligence in some manner.

In the immediate case, Fannie Fidget would be personally liable for her own negligent actions under the doctrine of personal liability and failure to act as a reasonably prudent nurse would act in applying hot water bottles. Healing Arts Hospital, as the employer of Fannie, would be vicariously liable under the doctrine of respondeat superior.

VIGNETTE 20

STAFFING

Susie Schzoid, R.N., was hired to work as a psychiatric nurse on the Psychiatric Unit and the mental health clinic at Healing Arts Hospital. On Tuesday morning Susie Schzoid arrived on duty at 8:00 A.M., according to hospital routine, and found she was scheduled to work with two patients admitted the night before. About 10 A.M. Clara Bartonette, supervisor, appeared on the unit and told Sally Schzoid it would be necessary for Sally to go to the Intensive Care Unit. Clara Bartonette explained to Sally that the Psychiatric Unit had excess staff. Simultaneously the Intensive Care Unit was understaffed because there were so many emergency admissions to the Intensive Care Unit during the night.

Susie Schzoid informs Clara Bartonette that she is unfamiliar with the Intensive Care Unit. Susie Schzoid further informs Clara Bartonette she feels she cannot give safe care to such ill patients.

What, if any, are the legal risks for Susie Schzoid and Clara Bartonette under these circumstances?

Answer

The first issue to be considered is what was the understanding between Susie Schzoid, R.N., and the hospital–employer upon her being hired. Was Susie hired specifically as a psychiatric nurse with the understanding that she would not be moved from floor to floor? There is a contract between Suzie Schzoid and Healing Arts Hospital. This contract may be implied or expressed. But the contract would be a composite of the understanding of the parties involved, any written documents, and the policies of the hospital. If a determination of the contract demonstrates that Susie Schzoid was hired as a psychiatric nurse, then Susie would be within her legal rights to refuse to go to the Intensive Cart Unit.

When a nurse is originally employed, there should be a clear understanding of mutual rights and responsibilities. The employer should make a determination of the education, skills, and experience possessed by the nurse and her level of patient care assignment should be made accordingly. If nursing service intends to move personnel from unit to unit, it should be made clear to the staff during the hiring process that this is the policy.

On the other hand hospitals cannot be economically or safely maintained if there is excess staff on one unit and insufficient staff on another unit.

Clara Bartonette did not describe the situation she was faced with as an emergency. If it were an emergency, Clara Bartonette could have asked Susie Schzoid to go to the Intensive Care Unit and do the best she could under the circumstances. For example, Susie Schzoid could be assigned care with another nurse rather than assigned to give medications.

At the same time, nursing staff should not refuse to go to another unit saying they are not capable of giving safe care when they simply do not want to go.

Hospitals should have continuing education programs where nursing staff can learn and maintain skills in giving patient care. It would be appropriate for nurses to be rotated through the various units when they can be taught at an appropriate pace. Thus staff can learn and be better utilized.

However the specific contract between Susie Schzoid and the hospital would take precedence in this case. Nursing service would be obliged to honor the contract made. Sally Schzoid would not be obligated to cover the Intensive Care Unit. It is the legal obligation of Clara Bartonette to see that the Intensive Care Unit has adequate coverage when circumstances increase patient occupancy.

VIGNETTE 21

COMMUNICATIONS

Vicky Vance, R.N., is the charge nurse in the emergency room. Clara Bartonette is the evening supervisor for several units including the emergency room at Healing Arts Hospital. On this particular weekend about 9:30 P.M., there is a multiple-car accident on the expressway near Healing Arts Hospital. The victims of the multiple-car accident are being brought into Healing Arts Hospital emergency room for treatment.

Newspaper reporters arrive at the hospital shortly after the victims. The newspaper reporters begin asking Vicky Vance a variety of questions about the victims. Several reporters are very aggressive and tell Vicky Vance the press has a right to know all about the victims. In fact they say they have an obligation to inform the public under "the public's right to know" doctrine. In addition, there are constant phone calls from persons inquiring about the identification and condition of the victims. Vicky Vance notifies Clara Bartonette, R.N., supervisor, of the situation and asks Clara Bartonette what information she may give to the inquiries being made.

What should Clara Bartonette's response be? What, if any, legal implications are involved?

Answer

Certain information is available and accessible for publication based on the following criteria.

A) It is a matter of public record and considered information accessible to the public domain.
B) It is a matter of concern or responsibility of civil authorities.
C) It is a matter involving a person of public interest or a public official.

Since the communications media consider such subjects as multiple accidents, gunshot wounds, or disaster-type episodes newsworthy, health care personnel should be prepared to handle such requests for information. The ideal situation is to have a public relations department available in each health agency to whom such issues may be referred. The realistic solution is to teach personnel how to handle such situations since some health care agencies do not have public relations personnel available on a 24 hour basis, if at all. Therefore, the evening supervisor who finds herself or himself in a "newsworthy situation" without appropriate available resources could utilize the following guidelines to avoid any legal risk.

It is always appropriate to get the permission of the patient and the attending physician before releasing any information; however, when this is impossible or impractical, the following information may be released: personal information such as name, address, age, sex, marital status; occupation may be made available and name of next-of-kin, if patient has expired. Only general information about the nature of the accident should be given, for example: "Car accident, the victim incurred internal injuries and was taken to shock trauma unit."

If the accident or injury involves shooting, mugging, knives, razors, or poisoning, it is considered a police matter and questions should be referred to the appropriate public or police authorities.

If the injury falls into the category of drug addiction, intoxication, attempted suicide, or suicide, no statements should be made related to these categories.

Finally, it is acceptable to make a general statement regarding the general condition of the patient such as there were minor injuries, internal injuries, third degree burns to face and arms, or condition is fair, satisfactory, or critical.

The issue is the patient's right to privacy and the public's right to know. The law has always attempted to protect the individual citizen's right to be free from unwarranted intrusion into their private lives. The Restatement of Torts, section 652A, recognizes a tort for invasion of privacy where there has been unreasonable intrusion on the seclusion of another. There is a general assumption at law that individual privacy must yield to the greater social benefits to be gained by the use of certain information about private individuals.

The guidelines previously suggested are based on patient information being classified as A) informational and non-confidential such as name, age, and occupation, and B) clinical and confidential, such as diagnosis, treatment, progress—the personal and private nature of data generally found in the clinical section of the medical record.

Although informational and non-confidential information can be released without the written consent of the patient, it should be done with care. The health care agency should have clearly defined policies and procedures on what may be disclosed and by whom.

VIGNETTE 22

PHARMACY

Patsy Peddler, R.N., is the charge nurse in the Coronary Care Unit at Healing Arts Hospital. She has been working the night shift on the unit for the past three months. One night about 2 A.M., Mrs. Rose Cardiac is admitted to the Coronary Care Unit. Her physician, Dr. Tachy, orders a heart stimulant to be given every four hours.

Patsy Peddler checks the medication supply and observes the drug is not available and it is not on the emergency drug cart or any other floors. Patsy Peddler checks the P.D.R. (Physician's Desk Reference) and finds that there is a drug available on the unit with the same pharmacologic properties. Patsy Peddler notifies Dr. Tachy that the drug ordered is not available. She also informs she checked the P.D.R. and there is a comparable drug on the floor and asks if Dr. Tachy wants to change the order.

Dr. Tachy insists that the specific drug he ordered for Mrs. Cardiac be given, and says, "Go to the pharmacy and get it."

What, if any, are the legal risks?

Answer

There is often a "practice gap" between the actions or scope of practice sanctioned by law and the actual practice expected by the health care practitioner in the daily work situation. Nowhere is this more true than on an evening or night shift where the nurse suddenly finds herself expected to assume the duties of certain disciplines that, although accessible on the day shift, are not accessible after 4 or 5 P.M. and on weekends.

Nurses on evening and night shifts, and especially those in a supervisory position, find themselves in the dilemma of practicing pharmacy without a license or sticking to the letter of the law, causing patients to go without necessary medications.

The pharmacy act states that it is the function of the pharmacist to identify, compound, package, dispense, label and preserve medications. It is clear that no one but a pharmacist may substitute for a pharmacist.

Nurses are licensed and authorized to administer medications, but are not authorized to dispense medications. That is the function of the pharmacist, and a nurse would be violating the Pharmacy Act and be guilty of an illegal act if she were to dispense medications. Drug administration is defined as the giving of a single dose of a medication to a patient pursuant to an order of a licensed medical doctor or other licensed practitioner, such as a dentist.

It therefore follows that it is an acceptable nursing function, within the legal parameters of the Pharmacy Act and considered drug administration, to remove from the pharmacy one dose of a particular drug for a particular patient.

There are unanticipated emergencies or contingencies that may occur with limited reaction time and resources available, such as in an emergency occurring in the early morning hours. Because of this, there should be a policy developed by an interdisciplinary committee with pharmacists, physicians, nurses, administrators, and other appropriate disciplines to create standard operating procedure for the nurse to follow. This committee should develop protocol, designate and authorize the appropriate person, for example, the night supervisor, to utilize the services of the pharmacy under certain conditions.

Some protocol provisions to be considered might include when the nurse may enter the pharmacy under "certain conditions." It is suggested that the pharmacist provide an emergency pharmaceutical kit containing those drugs which are necessary for the particular needs of the hospital during the interim when the pharmacist is absent from the hospital. The necessary records should be kept indicating the drug removed, the exact dosage, the purpose or patient for whom the drug was removed and the nurse's signature.

If a drug is ordered and it is not available in the emergency pharmaceutical kit or not available for any other reasons, the pharmacist designated for such occasions should be notified and should provide the necessary emergency service of dispensing the required medication.

This is not an unusual situation, and when such situations tend to repeat themselves, no nurse should permit herself to be put at legal risk. Common sense and the reasonably prudent nurse would take the necessary action to insure that they are authorized to act in the patient's best interest by getting the specific medication ordered for the patient's health care. She should assure that she acts in her own best interest by being covered by, and following, policy developed by the hospital interdisciplinary committee.

VIGNETTE 23

PROTECTING PERSONAL PROPERTY

Clara Bartonette is the night supervisor in a small community hospital having 150 beds. Mrs. Marie Watcher comes to the emergency room complaining of vomiting and diarrhea at approximately 1:00 A.M. The patient is examined and routinely admitted to the hospital as an inpatient with the tentative diagnosis of food poisoning. The patient, Mrs. Marie Watcher, is transferred to the medical floor with her clothing and personal effects. At approximately 2:30 A.M., after Mrs. Marie Watcher is placed in bed and while the nurse is taking her T.P.R. and blood pressure, she states the diamond wedding ring she had on her left hand is missing. She also says the ring is worth $500 and she wants it back immediately or she is going to sue the nurse and the hospital for negligence in caring for her and her property.

> Who, if anyone, is liable? What principles of law, if any, are involved?
> Is the hospital responsible for the patient's property?
> Would there be a different outcome if the patient were unconscious?

Answer

It is general policy in most health care agencies to have available a place for safe keeping of any valuable articles. Upon admission the patient should be asked if she has any valuables that she would want placed in the hospital safe. If there are family present, the patient should be given the option of entrusting any valuables to the family. The hospital and the nursing personnel have an obligation to exercise reasonable care in protecting the patient's money and valuables. Reasonable care requires that the hospital provide a safe place and notify the patient of the opportunity to place valuables there.

But the hospital or nursing personnel are not guarantors that the patient's possessions will not be stolen. They only promise to provide reasonable security. The patient was conscious when admitted and in control of all her faculties. She was aware of the ring and the value. Therefore, it was incumbent on the patient to take ordinary precaution to protect her possessions. The patient has a duty to act as a reasonably prudent person at all times. It would seem the prudent thing to do, to take the precaution to notify the hospital personnel of the ring and the approximate value and request the article be placed in a safe.

When property is entrusted to the hospital for safekeeping, a bailment relationship takes place. Bailment is delivering of personal property to another for a specific purpose. The bailor is the person who delivers the property. The bailee is the one to whom the property is delivered. When the purpose for the bailment is achieved, the bailee returns the article to the bailor. The bailee must take reasonable care of the property entrusted and is liable for loss or damage to the property caused by bailee's negligence.

The nurse should make the necessary documentations and have a witness verify the specific amount, if money is involved, and the specific article if rings, watches, or other valuable articles are involved.

If the patient is unconscious, the nurse would have a higher duty to protect the patient's possessions. On admission to any unit, part of the admission procedure should be a protocol for covering patient's belongings. The observant nurse will consider patient's possessions as part of the general assessment made at the time of admission and follow procedure.

However, if articles are missing from the patient and the nurse had no knowledge of the incident neither the nurse nor the hospital will be held liable. The standard of care is ordinary reasonable care and as long as the nurse acts as a reasonably prudent nurse would act in the same circumstances, she has met the standard expected.

When the patient is admitted to the hospital he often brings several types of property with him. There is property having a monetary value, that is, money, rings, or watches. There is property of a personal nature such as false teeth, eye glasses, contact lenses or other prostheses. There is property having a religious or sentimental value such as a Bible, medals, or crosses.

It is incumbent on the hospital and the hospital administrator to maintain an environment of safety and security for the patient and the patient's property. The law applied here is that of bailment. The patient has a right to expect that any property entrusted to the hospital's care through the agency of the personnel working there will be returned intact. The hospital administration is not responsible for any property of which it had no knowledge. However, if any property which has been deposited for safekeeping is damaged or missing, the hospital would be liable.

There are certain precautions regarding property that reasonably prudent patients should take. Patients are bound by the reasonably prudent man doctrine. Therefore, the patient should not bring valuable property to a health care agency, since no health care agency can guarantee that nothing will happen to property in the complicated matrix system of a hospital. If the patient is admitted under circumstances in which he could not foresee or make preparations for the valuables on him, the valuables should be given to a spouse, or member of the family, with appropriate documentation of the event, such as a receipt from the family member.

VIGNETTE 24

WILLS

Fannie Funnie is a private duty nurse. She has worked in various hospitals in the state for over 15 years doing private duty. Presently, she works for the Central Registry affiliated with the State Nurses Association.

For the past several weeks, she has been doing special duty at the Healing Arts Hospital. She has been caring for Mr. Heartley, a 55-year-old man who has undergone heart by-pass surgery for a condition involving atherosclerosis.

One particular evening, Mr. Heartley is very depressed. He begins to talk about death and dying. After a period of time, Mr. Heartley asks Fanny Funnie to call an attorney. He wants to make his will. He asks her to be one of the witnesses when he signs the will. He also asks her to get whatever other witnesses are necessary to make the will a valid document. He says his attorney will explain all that, but could he depend on her to get the necessary witnesses, because it is late evening and he does not want to disturb his family or upset them that he is making a will.

Fanny Funnie has never been in this type of situation before. She is perplexed and does not know what to do.

What, if anything, should Fanny Funnie do?
What, if any, are the legal risks involved if she calls an attorney?

What, if any, are the legal risks involved if she does not call an attorney?

Should Fannie Funnie witness the will as requested by Mr. Heartley? Why or why not?

Answer

It has been the experience of the authors in speaking with health care professionals that they are extremely reluctant to witnesss any legal documents and in particular a last will and testament of a patient. It is true that there is no legal obligation to witness any such documents, but it would seem there is certainly a strong moral and ethical obligation. If one reflects on this issue, what is more important than the patient's peace of mind? Where an individual has accumulated an estate throughout a lifetime, be it large or small, he wishes that estate to go to his loved ones or those he deems in need. Where the estate is one of sentimental value rather than monetary munificence, it is even more important to the testator (one making a will) that the articles of sentimental value go to the persons of his choosing.

But you will say, as has been said, "Suppose the lawyer's a crook or the family is forcing the patient to make a will." That would seem to be an even more important reason for you to witness the actual signing by the patient-testator. You could serve as an objective witness.

Many people postpone making a will and often the delay results in loss of assets to the very persons for whom the protection was intended. The main purpose of a will is to: 1) insure the assets are distributed as intended and 2) avoid unnecessary financial intanglement and taxation.

By making a will, the testator (one who makes a will) clearly defines his wishes and prevents ambiguities or misinterpretations. There are tragic examples of property being allowed to devolve legally according to a state's intestacy succession, but not morally, because no will was made. The law is dynamic. One should remember that subsequent laws may be enacted to change present intestacy laws.

The health care professional is not going to assist in drawing up the will, or performing any arts of legal assistance. That could be construed as practicing law without a license. The role of the health care professional is to witness the act of the testator signing the document as his last will and testament—to witness that, at this time to the best of your knowledge, the testator was of sound mind, was lucid, and understood the effect of the acts he was performing. You would be witnessing that the testator was under no overt coercion, and as far as you could ascertain, was performing the act freely, willingly, and under his own impetus.

Everyday, health care professionals make notations on a patient's chart of what they perceive through their senses regarding a patient's condition and reaction to drugs and procedures. There is no reluctance to this form of record keeping. Possibly the reason is that this action is seen as a traditional function and witnessing wills or other legal documents is not.

It should be clear to the health care professional that as a witness to the will, there is no attesting to the wisdom of the testator's choices. A witness does not have to second guess the testator or in any way give counsel or advice. It would be inappropriate to do so and might be construed as the practice of law if a health care professional should attempt to offer legal advice. The health care professional can best serve the patient's need in this respect by simply observing all the circumstances under which the will was signed and be prepared to testify to the observations made.

This service for the patient should be fully appreciated. It is just as important to witness a document for the patient which the patient has requested as it is to give the right medication, or treatment. This will is the most important legal document a person will execute to provide for his family or dependents. What will be the alternative if a patient is unable to execute a proper will because he was unable to get witnesses to attest to the signing? If an individual dies without making a will, the distribution of the individual's estate will be by intestacy or intestate succession. This is a distribution made by the state according to a particular schedule. This schedule which would be implemented in lieu of a will, generally would not be the testator's choice had a will been made.

Also, the testator may wish to reject entirely or revise partially a previous will. This option should be available to the patient at all times.

Health professionals also argue that the patient should have had his will made out prior to coming to the health care center. There is no quarreling with that statement. Unfortunately, humans tend to procrastinate over making wills. Death is not a subject that is easily faced, and avoidance of making a will so closely connected with one's demise is understandable, but not condonable. How often do members of the legal profession die intestate? These professionals, more than any other persons, should appreciate the necessity of a will to avoid delay and complications for loved ones.

It is for the reasons stated and others not stated because they would involve a treatise on testamentary law, that a patient should be assisted in every way if he wishes to make a last will and testament.

As stated, the will is the legal document which will protect the patient's loved ones following his demise. It is well to have an understanding of the law regarding wills to better serve the patient and one's self.

A will according to Black's *Law Dictionary* is the "the legal expression or declaration of a person's mind or wishes" as to the disposition of his property to be performed or take effect after his death. There are certain elements or conditions that must be met to ensure that a will is valid at law. First, the testator must have testamentary capacity. By testamentary capacity is meant that the testator understands and appreciates the significance of his actions. For example, the testator knows what his assets are and knows the disposition he is about to make of those assets to the appropriate persons of his choice. Therefore, it follows that a patient must be mentally competent, he cannot be under the influence of drugs or alcohol to the extent that he is unable to appreciate his actions. But the mere fact that the patient has had some medication or some wine or alcohol does not destroy his testamentary capacity. The test to determine if the patient has the necessary capacity is his ability to understand and appreciate his actions. If that test is met, then that particular element or condition is met.

A second element or condition is that the testator declare or tell the witnesses that the document or instrument is his will and he wishes them to witness his signature to that document. It is not necessary for the witnesses to have any knowledge of the contents of the will.

There are certain formalities governed by statute in each state. This is the attorney's responsibility to see that those formalities are met. If the health care professional accepts the responsibility of being a witness to a will or any legal document, then the responsibility is to assist the testator in any appropriate manner by fulfilling any reasonable requests in this regard. It is also appropriate and prudent for the health care professional to record the event of the execution of the will, the mental and physical condition of the patient, the names of the witnesses to the event and any other information deemed significant.

The health care professional can play an important role in the patient's health care by taking a positive attitude when called upon to witness any legal documents. It is hoped that this explanation will alert health care professionals to the significance of their actions and the effect of any inaction on the patient while alive and on the patient's family when he is dead.

VIGNETTE 24 A

WILLS—SIGNATURE

Dottie Doubtful, R.N., is a private duty nurse. She has worked in various hospitals in the state for over 15 years. Presently, she is working for the Central Registry affiliated with the State Nurses' Association. For the past several weeks, she has been working at Healing Arts Hospital. She is taking care of Mr. Blalock. He is a 72-year-old diabetic with blindness in both eyes as a result of retinal neuropathy. He has also had a cardiovascular accident and is partially paralyzed on his right side and has difficulty using his right arm. Mr. Blalock informs Dottie he wants to rescind his old will and write a new one. He wants to leave a large bequest to Healing Arts Hospital. He asks Dottie to call his attorney and to serve as a witness to his last will and testament.

Dottie has never been in this type of situation. She is willing to be a witness for Mr. Blalock. But Dottie Doubtful is unsure of the legal implications. Since Mr. Blalock is blind and paralyzed and unable to sign his name to a legal document, Dottie is concerned he would not have the necessary testamentary capacity.

What, if anything, should be done in this situation?

Answer

If a testator is unable to sign his name because of illiteracy, physical weakness or other similar condition, the testator may affix his mark normally with an X and have one or both witnesses identify it in the following manner.

Billy Blalock

His

X

Mark

In the present case, Mr. Blalock is blind but literate; that is, he has the intellectual ability to read but lacks the physical capacity to do so. It would be perfectly legal and proper for one of the witnesses to assist Mr. Blalock and guide his hand in signing the will. All witnesses to the will should be present at the same time when the testator executes (that is, makes his mark and has his hand guided) the will. This is a perfectly legitimate procedure. The issue is that the testator fully understands that his or her signature is being affixed to the will. The fact that the testator is being assisted by another party does not diminish his legal and testamentary capacity.

VIGNETTE 25

INSURANCE SITUATION

Sara Gampie, R.N., is a staff nurse working in the emergency room. She has been working in the unit for six months. Previously, Sara Gampie was on a Medical-Surgical Unit. Sara Gampie returned from a committee meeting very upset one morning.

The committee was discussing the implication of risk management data for the past six months in the Healing Arts Hospital. The committee had been established to deal with the malpractice and liability problems throughout the hospital. The data revealed that the emergency room had the highest number of incidents involving some type of patient injury compared to any unit in the hospital. Sara Gampie told Clara Bartonette, R.N., supervisor, of her concern regarding the committee's data. This data included all the incidents that had occurred throughout the hospital. Sara Gampie stated she did not have any personal liability malpractice insurance and was afraid of being sued while working as an emergency room nurse.

Clara Bartonette, supervisor, responds to Sara Gampie by telling Sara, "There is no need to worry, I have asked Ms. Prudence Pumpernickel, Director of Nurses, about the situation. Ms. Pumpernickel has reassured me on several occasions that the hospital insurance policy covers all the employees and this includes all the nurses; so there is no need to worry." Prudence had received this information from the hospital attorney.

> Sara Gampie still has concern over the situation; what, if anything, should she do?
> What, if any, legal implications should Sara Gampie be aware of?

Answer

Today we are all concerned about insurance. It is the civilized method of distributing risk. Most of us pay required premiums for health insurance, car insurance, life insurance and home insurance.

In fact, if one wanted—or could afford—to deal with Lloyds of London, one could have his hands or voice or any precious possession insured for a sufficient premium.

Insurance is a contract or agreement by which an insurer agrees to assume certain risks of the insured for a premium. The insurer agrees to pay the insured, or certain persons, a specific amount of money if the event for which insurance has been taken occurs.

Insurance policies are usually elaborate, as most laymen know. In fact, lawyers, with tongue in cheek, advise that the best way of reviewing a policy is just to read the fine print. So, although an insurance policy may contain a great deal of extraneous material, there are certain necessary elements one should look for in any policy. The insurance policy will contain the identification of the risk involved, the specified occurence, and the specific amount payable should the event occur.

When analyzing an insurance policy, there are five distinct parts one should always review to have a better understanding of the actual coverage he has. The insurance agreement states what the insurer assumes to pay, or his legal liability, not any moral obligations. There is the policy period which clearly states that certain period of time when the policy is to be effective. There is a defense and settlement clause which defines how the company will defend the insured against suit and its power to settle claims against the insured. The policy will have a clause stating the amount of money the insurer will pay, how it will pay it, the maximum amounts it will pay. Finally, and one of the most important sections of the policy, are the conditions under which the policy will be paid. There are always important conditions in each liability contract, and failure to comply with those stated conditions could result in the policy's being forfeited or cancelled. An insurance policy is a contract with legal obligations on both sides between the insured and the insurer. Failure to meet those conditions by either party is a breach of the contract.

By risk one means there is a possibility some type of loss may occur. There are generally three categories of risk to which an individual is exposed. There is the risk to property where one incurs loss or damage; there is the risk to person, such as injury to health or life; and there is the risk to one's profession or legal liability, such as malpractice.

Insurance protection starts immediately when the agent gives the insured a binder. If no binder has been obtained from the agent, the insurance is generally not effective until the policy is delivered to the insured.

Obviously, it is difficult for the average person or family to bear the cost of serious damage to health, property, or person. Insurance is based on the principle that categories of persons exposed to the same type of risk or hazard pay premiums into a general fund from which the insured will be indemnified in the event the risk event occurs.

The professional liability insurance policies give standard coverage using a clause such as "to pay on behalf of the insured all sums which the insured shall become legally obligated to pay as damages because of injury arising out of malpractice, error or mistake in rendering or failing to render nursing services."

Do health professionals need to carry their own malpractice insurance? The answer, of course, depends on many factors that can only be judged by the individual health professional who can weigh all the factors and make an intelligent decision. However, the writer wishes to point out that few, if any, persons today would be without health insurance or automobile insurance. The risk involved in being without coverage is frightening to us all. We are all aware of persons who did not have adequate health coverage and whose financial resources were wiped out by lengthy illness. So, it would seem well worth the small premium for health professionals (excluding doctors) to carry professional liability insurance.

At present the average malpractice insurance premiums for health professionals cost about twelve dollars a year. That seems a small price to pay for peace of mind. Another observation is that as long as one finds the premiums so low, it indicates that the lawsuits are not numerous. It is logical to assume that there is a direct relationship between the cost of the premium and the risks involved.

Why do health professionals need individual professional liability insurance? There is no assurance that a health professional will not be sued individually even though covered or partially covered by the hospital or agency for whom he works. Also, even though the employer may be liable under the doctrine of respondeat superior for the actions of the health professional, the employer, through his insurance company, may file a claim against the health professional to get back the money paid out. This is called subrogating the claim. The insurance company "stands in the shoes" of the employer. In fact, most insurance policies contain a subrogation clause which permits the insurance company to sue appropriate parties to regain any monies paid out under the insurance agreement. As stated elsewhere, the health professional can always be held liable for his own acts, whether named alone or as a co-defendant.

Malpractice liability insurance pays the court-awarded verdict, and the cost of legal counsel. If you procure a $50,000/$150,000 policy, this means your insurance company will pay a maximum of $50,000 in damages to any one person injured as a result of your malpractice and it will pay a maximum of $150,000 in damages in any one year on all claims against the health professional.

Health care is a high-risk area for most of us. With advanced technology, educated patients, and increased risks of lawsuits, the health practitioner must be fully aware of what coverage he has and what coverage he needs to be adequately protected in the event he must defend himself in a lawsuit.

The malpractice risk for health practitioners is significant and recent indications are that the risks will increase in importance. Practically all persons involved in the health field face the risk of a malpractice suit. A majority of health professionals recognize the significance of the risk exposure; those who have not done so should objectively examine their potential risk. The amount and limits of malpractice insurance should be commensurate with the risk of the health professional or hospital or health agency.

VIGNETTE 26

TEACHING CARDIOPULMONARY RESUSCITATION TO L.P.N.'S AND AIDES

Sara Gampie, R.N., is the charge nurse in the Coronary Care Unit. She has been working in the unit for a total of three years. The Coronary Care Unit has a capacity of 10 patients with corresponding emergency equipment for each patient's unit. Over this time, Sara Gampie has established the staffing pattern on each shift to include one to two licensed practical nurses and one to two nursing assistants as well as registered nurses. All the registered nurses have been trained in cardiopulmonary resuscitation.

The patients in this unit often go into cardiac arrest. There is monitoring equipment that buzzes when the patient's vital signs deviate abnormally and become life threatening. There is also an established protocol to follow under such circumstances.

On several occasions the licensed practical nurses and nursing assistants have complained that they do not know what to do in an emergency situation and want to receive training. Sara Gampie has reservations about anyone other than physicians or registered nurses performing cardiopulmonary resuscitation. The licensed practical nurses and nursing assistants have made a formal request in writing to Clara Bartonette, Supervisor, to receive training in cardiopulmonary resuscitation. Clara Bartonette has reviewed the entire situation with

Sara Gampie and has requested Sara to make a recommendation to Nursing Service Administration regarding this issue.

What, if any, recommendation would be appropriate for Sara Gampie, R.N., to make?
What, if any, rationale should be the basis for the recommendation?

Answer

In an emergency where life is endangered, anyone can do anything reasonably calculated to save the life of another. Therefore, it would seem reasonable to extend this fundamental legal maxim to give proper training to appropriate personnel who may be in a position to resuscitate a patient when a skilled physician is not available. It also follows that there should be a period of academic training and skill performance with a specific curriculum including performance and evaluation testing. Successful completion of the specified program could result in the trainee receiving a certificate. Certification is a process by which the agency or health institution grants recognition or acknowledges that an individual has satisfactorily completed certain predetermined qualifications or requisites. These qualifications or requisites have been identified by the health institution or agency as minimum standards to be met by any individual for certification. This certification process establishes a standardization for the organization, and for the individuals in the organization.

No health care practitioner should assume they have a monopoly on medical knowledge. Lay people are taking courses in emergency first aid and cardiopulmonary resuscitation. It is becoming a common procedure. It is important for all personnel in a unit such as emergency room, Coronary Care, or Intensive Care to be able to perform all necessary functions in emergencies to aid patients. No one can be certain when such a need will arise and a person trained to react appropriately is obviously in a better position to save a patient's life.

VIGNETTE 27

LABOR RELATIONS SITUATION

Carrie Crockett, R.N., is a supervisor at Healing Arts Hospital, Incorporated. She has worked on the 11:00 to 7:00 shift for five years; the 3:00 to 11:00 shift for five years; and is presently on the 7:00 to 3:00

shift. As part of her responsibilities, she supervises the Intensive Care Unit, the Coronary Care Unit, and the Shock Trauma Emergency Units. She is an experienced supervisor, respected by the employees and has a reputation for dealing fairly with all the employees when disciplining, hiring, firing, or performing any supervisory functions.

Carrie Crockett has been a member of the State Nurses' Association since graduating from Healing Arts Hospital School of Nursing 15 years ago. She has been an active member serving on several committees from time to time. Carrie feels a strong loyalty to both her State Nurses' Association and her employer, Healing Arts Hospital, Incorporated.

There has been increased organizational and union activity in recent years at Healing Arts Hospital and other hospitals in the surrounding areas. There have been indications that the AFL-CIO union, the Teamsters, and the State Nurses' Association are actively campaigning to persuade the employees to vote for their particular group as the exclusive bargaining agent for Healing Arts Hospital and the nearby area hospitals.

Carrie Crockett is essentially an anti-union person. However, she believes the State Nurses' Association would be the most acceptable group to represent the nurses in the hospital if there must be such activity. Carrie Crockett contacts the chairman of the organizing committee at the State Nurses' Association and agrees to assist the committee in signing up the registered nurses at Healing Arts Hospital to petition the employer to recognize the State Nurses' Association as the exclusive bargaining agent. Carrie Crockett makes it very clear to the committee she will not put any pressure on any of the nurses to sign up. Her role will be only one of assistance to facilitate their choice of the State Nurses' Association.

Carrie Crockett begins to function in the above manner. After three days of such activity, she is charged with participating in an unfair labor practice. She denies the charges; what, if any, is the liability?

Healing Arts Hospital, Incorporated, is also charged with unfair labor practices. The hospital denies liability, stating the hospital had absolutely no knowledge of Carrie Crockett's activity and even if they did, they were not responsible for such activity, that Carrie alone should be held personally liable. What result?

Answer

The first issue is to determine if Carrie Crockett is a supervisor as defined by the National Labor Relations Board. According to the board, a supervisor is one who has the responsibility of directing the work of others and who has the authority to affect the status of employees. That is "any individual having authority, in the interest of the employer, to hire, transfer, suspend, lay off, recall, promote, discharge, assign, reward, or discipline other employees, responsible for directing them, adjust their grievances, or effectively to recommend such action, if in connection with the foregoing the exercise of such authority is not of a merely routine or clerical nature, but requires the use of independent judgment." Carrie Crockett meets this criteria and is therefore designated a supervisor.

The next issue is the question of Carrie's activities on behalf of the State Nurses' Association. It is clear from the facts that Carrie is in no way interfering with any of the other union's activities. She also acted in good faith, believing her professional organization to be the most competent to work for the best interests of the nurses and the patients. Nevertheless this can be considered an unfair labor practice.

The procedure in an unfair labor practice case is begun by any person filing a charge with the regional office. The charge must be signed, sworn to or affirmed under oath. The charged party is notified of the charges and the time of a hearing to answer the charges. The fact that Carrie had no intention of influencing any nurses improperly, the fact that Carrie only intended to do what she believed in the best interests of the patients, would be irrelevant. Section 8 (B) (1) (A) of the NLR Act forbids conduct that independently restrains or coerces employees. It does not matter how successful or how subtle that activity. It could still be construed as an unfair labor practice. In this instance, Carrie's activity could be interpreted by the board as a subtle intimidation of nurse employees to join the group being assisted by Carrie.

It is an unfair labor practice for a supervisor to actively participate in efforts to form or assume any administrative role in a union seeking to represent non-supervisory employees.

The third issue is that Carrie is a supervisor. As such, she is part of management. This means that her activity in this case is imputed to the employer. The fact that the employer did not know of the activity and did not condone the activity, is irrelevant. One of the purposes of the National Labor Relations act is to protect employees from the unfair labor practices of employers, and to protect the rights of employees from practices that are harmful to the general welfare. A supervisor is an agent of management. A supervisor acts in the interest of the employer. Therefore, it is as though the employer were itself performing the improper activity. Therefore, the Healing Arts Hospital, Incorporated, would be liable for any unfair labor practice engaged in by agent-supervisor, Carrie Crockett.

VIGNETTE 28

WORKMEN'S COMPENSATION CASE

Margy Magg, R.N., was lifting a patient onto a stretcher following a call from the X-ray department. Ms. Magg felt something snap in her back, and a pain shot down her left leg. She continued to work although she was in severe pain. The charge nurse advised Ms. Magg to go to the health clinic to be examined. Following a visit to the health clinic, X-rays of Margy Magg's back were taken. The X-ray revealed a herniated lumbar intervertebral disc between the fourth and fifth lumbar vertebra. There were also arthritic, degenerative disc changes.

Margy Magg filed a workmen's compensation claim alleging the above facts and claiming that she was injured in the line of duty. The employer-hospital denied the allegations, stating there was a prior injury which caused the plaintiff's backache and disability. The hospital also argued the registered nurse should have sought help in moving the patient. Even if the nurse did injure herself as she alleged, it could have been prevented by acting as a reasonably prudent nurse and seeking assistance.

What decision should be made in this case and why?

Answer

The facts of the case show that Margy Magg was injured while on duty and while caring for a patient. The key test is that the injuries arose out of and in the course of her employment. Nurse Margy Magg followed appropriate procedure and hospital policy following the injury. She dutifully reported the injury, underwent examination and X-rays.

The purpose of workmen's compensation insurance is to protect workers who were injured on the job. It is not a question of assigning negligence or assessing wrongdoing. Workmen's compensation benefits should be awarded to the nurse or any other employee injured in the course of their employment.

VIGNETTE 29

POLICE POWERS SITUATION

Myrtle Medic, R.N., is a staff nurse working for a public health agency for several years. She works in a specific community area and is assigned a specific number of patients in a census tract as her caseload. As part of her caseload, she carries the Carroll family. The Carroll family consists of Mr. and Mrs. Carroll, a son, Tommie, 14 years old, and a daughter, Jane, who is 10 years old. Jane has been hospitalized recently. Myrtle Medic receives a call from the charge nurse at Happy Hills Hospital requesting a written appraisal of the Carroll home situation. This request is being made because Jane Carroll is being discharged following treatment for tuberculosis. The appraisal is to determine the adequacy and suitability of the home and the parents to competently care for the patient following discharge.

> Does Nurse Myrtle Medic have to get permission from the parents to assess the home situation or to give such assessment to the charge nurse requesting it, from Happy Hills Hospital?
> Would Nurse Medic be at legal risk for her actions or inactions in such a situation?

Answer

There is an important constitutional right given to the states called "Police Power." Under Police Power, the states have the obligation and duty to protect the health and welfare of their citizens. This Police Power is generally delegated to a specific health agency by the governor or legislature of a particular state. In most states, this agency is known as the public health department. It is as the name implies—charged with maintaining the public health. In order to maintain the public health, certain powers are necessary. These certain powers to do what is needed to be done are inherent in the delegation of Police Powers. The public health officer can go so far as to order the arrest of an individual who has a communicable disease and refuses treatment, thereby subjecting all the citizens to the potential risk of contracting the communicable disease. It is also the Police Power that permits states to require licenses of certain classes of professions that deal in the public sector; example, beauticians, doctors, nurses, barbers, electricians, and whoever may affect the public health.

The public health nurse has delegated authority to carry out the purposes of the public health department. In the instant case, a ten-year-old child with tuberculosis is a potentially contaminating and infectious individual. The public health nurse, as a matter of courtesy, should contact the parents or guardian and make arrangements to visit and appraise the home. As a matter of law, however, the public health nurse would have the right under the authority delegated to her through the Police Powers of the state to enter the house and make the appropriate appraisal.

In many states, there is also a visiting nurses' association. These associations are sometimes a combined public health–visiting nurse association. In other states there is a separate and distinct visiting nurses' association which is non-profit. In those instances where the visiting nurses' association is called upon to make such home appraisals as described in the previous vignette, there is a clear distinction.

The instructive visiting nurses' association or similar association is a non-profit organization created by a charter given by the secretary of state of the particular state in which the organization is founded. Although the organization is dedicated to the health and welfare of the citizens of the particular state, it has no authority under the Police Power of the state. Therefore, the visiting nurse would not have the same right as that delegated by the public health agency to enter a home uninvited or unauthorized. It would be clearly necessary for the visiting nurse to seek and receive the permission of the parents or guardian or owners of the home to which the child is being discharged before attempting to make an appraisal.

This is an interesting example of the distinction in authority between two agencies where all facts are the same—the staff apparently with similar qualifications, yet with a different authorization and legal power.

VIGNETTE 30

CONTRIBUTORY NEGLIGENCE OR COMPARATIVE NEGLIGENCE SITUATION

John Heartache was a 60-year-old male with the diagnosis of congestive heart failure. He was mentally alert. But he would doze frequently as a result of medications given for anxiety he was experiencing. John Heartache was a chain smoker. He smoked incessantly and said he would not and could not curtail his smoking. Medical orders included oxygen p.r.N. as part of the plan of care. The patient was instructed not to smoke and to wear hospital pajamas to avoid static electricity. Notations on the nursing care plan said, "Remove all cigarettes, matches, and lighters from the patient and patient's night stand."

One evening around 10:00 P.M., the evening supervisor smelled smoke. Upon entering Mr. Heartache's room, the supervisor found the bed on fire. Mr. Heartache suffered third degree burns of the arms and face and first degree burns of his chest.

Mr. Heartache sued the evening staff and the hospital, alleging negligence. He said it was foreseeable the patient could have been burned under these circumstances. The patient plaintiff also alleged the staff and hospital had not taken sufficient measures to protect him, that a duty of due care was owed by the hospital and the duty was breached and the breach was the proximate cause of John Heartache's burns. The hospital denies all charges.

What, if any, liability is there for the staff and hospital? Why?

Answer

The cause of the fire was not established. The staff had followed hospital policy. The staff instructed Mr. Heartache not to smoke and to use only hospital gowns. He was mentally competent and capable of protecting himself. On the other hand, the staff should take precautionary measures and remove all flammable materials from Mr. Heartache. The staff should see that there are sufficient hospital pajamas so the patient would not be tempted to use non-hospital pajamas. This case could be a question of fact for the jury. Where there is contradictory evidence regarding the question of due care, the jury may be called upon to decide the issue. The jury would decide if the staff and hospital, under these particular facts and circumstances, did everything reasonably expected of them to protect the patient. If the answer is yes, there would be no liability. The second issue would be to determine if the patient acted as a reasonably prudent patient would act under similar circumstances or did the patient contribute to his own injury? The answer to that question would determine liability. If the patient persisted in smoking or wearing a non-hospital gown and a fire resulted, the patient would be negligent and the cause of his own injury. No recovery could occur under those circumstances.

In states which recognize the doctrine of contributory negligence, the argument would be that John Heartache contributed to his own negligence by not acting as a reasonably prudent patient and causing injury to himself. If these facts were proven, there would be no recovery for John Heartache.

In states which recognize the doctrine of comparative negligence, there would be the argument that although Mr. Heartache was the cause of some injury to himself, the hospital, through its staff, was also the proximate cause of those injuries. If the facts are proven and accepted by a jury, there would be an assessment of damages.

In this particular case, the court ruled that the hospital and staff were not liable for Mr. Heartaches' injury.

VIGNETTE 31

MEDICATION ADMINISTRATION

Linda Lacey, R.N., is a recent graduate from Clara Barton Community College Associate Degree Program. She has begun working at Healing Arts Hospital, Incorporated, and has been working there for six months. The first three months, Linda Lacey was assigned to the Medical-Surgical unit for orientation. She has been through the probation period required by the hospital policy which is a six-month period.

Linda Lacey has been assigned to give all medication, including injections, to the patients on the Medical-Surgical unit. There are 35 patients on this particular unit.

While giving medications, she receives a phone call from Dr. Sam Scapel. Dr. Scapel tells Linda Lacey, R.N., to give Mrs. Nellie Nervosa, his private patient, who is a post-operative gastrectomy, Dramamine for nausea. Dr. Scapel tells Ms. Lacey, R.N., to write the order as "Dramamine 75 mg hypodermically Q 4 H PRN." Shortly after Dr. Scapel calls, Mrs. Nervosa asks for some medication to relieve her nausea. She has had no other medications for over six hours.

Linda Lacey administered the injection of Dramamine subcutaneously in the left arm of the patient. Mrs. Nervosa developed a hard reddened inflamed area over the injection site. The patient complained of pain and limitation of arm movement. Dr. Scapel was notified of the situation. He examined Mrs. Nervosa's left arm and diagnosed the developing lump as a fat necrosis of the tissue due to trauma.

Who, if anyone, would be liable in these circumstances?

Answer

Dramamine in hypodermic form is a drug which should be given intramuscularly for better and proper absorption. A Dramamine injection is irritating in the tissues and can cause injury or, as happened in this case, necrosis.

The nurse did not act appropriately for several reasons. Linda Lacey gave the injection without a clear route of administration. "Hypodermically" can mean either subcutaneously or intramuscularly. In this particular set of facts, the method of injection made a significant difference. Nurses are expected to be familiar with the medications they administer. It is also incumbent upon them as professionals to make certain judgments and to interpret the doctor's orders according to the skill, training, and experience of comparable registered nurses. If the nurse had any doubt what Dr. Scapel meant by hypodermic, that is, if the route were to be intramuscular or subcutaneous, the doubt should have been resolved before Linda Lacey proceeded.

Nurses are expected to carry out the physician's orders without causing injury to the patient. Linda Lacey also failed to meet the standard of care reasonably prudent nurses in the same set of circumstances are expected to meet. In this situation, Linda Lacey was expected to know that an irritating medication injected subcutaneously could cause irritation and consequent injury at the site of injection.

Linda Lacey's negligence is very clear. She has a duty of care to Mrs. Nervosa. The duty was breached by giving the medication improperly. Mrs. Nervosa was injured as a result, and the proximate cause of injury was the act of Linda Lacey. There was a definite causal connection between the injury and the negligence of Linda Lacey.

Linda Lacey would generally be liable for the patient's injury under the doctrine of personal liability. The Healing Arts Hospital would generally be liable under the doctrine of respondeat superior because Linda Lacey was an employee of the hospital and she was working within the scope of her authority when the injury to the patient took place.

VIGNETTE 32

SEARCH AND SEIZURE

Sarah Gampie, R.N., was working in the emergency room on the 3:00 to 11:00 P.M. shift. The emergency room was unusually busy this particular evening. Two patients, both male, Jesse and Jeffrey James, each 22 years old, were brought to Healing Arts Hospital, Incorporated, emergency room by two police officers, one of whom was a police sergeant. The sergeant said he wanted to talk with the doctor regarding the two patients just admitted. Sergeant Edgett Hoover then told the doctor on duty, Dr. Kris Kritical, he was to do a blood alcohol and a blood barbiturate on both patients. Sergeant Edgett Hoover then asked the nurse, Sarah Gampie, to search the clothes and belongings of Jesse and Jeffrey James to locate any narcotics they are believed to have in their possession.

Sarah Gampie, R.N., and Kris Kritical, M.D., want to be cooperative with the police officers, but are not sure what legal risks are involved.

1. Should Kris Kritical draw blood on Jesse and Jeffrey

James as requested by the police officers?
Would there be any liability?

2. Should Sarah Gampie comply with the request to search
for drugs the patients may have in their possession?
What, if any, legal liability could result?

Answer

The Fourth Amendment to the Constitution of the United States
states, "the right of the people to be secure in their persons, houses,
papers, and effects, against unreasonable searches and seizures shall
not be violated, and no warrants shall issue, but *upon probable cause*,
supported by oath or affirmation, and particularly describing the place
to be searched, and the persons or things to be seized. The Constitution of the United States confers certain rights on all its citizens. The
fourth amendment confers the right to be left alone, to be free from
warrantless intrusions, to have privacy, to be secure in one's person
and one's personal effects. This is not an absolute right but is a qualified right. This qualified personal right must yield to society's greater
right. This means the fourth amendment does not confer an absolute
right of prohibiting all searches and seizures. It gives the protection
of a qualified right and prohibits all unreasonable searches of a person
or a person's personal effects.

In the Landmark case of *Mapp v. Ohio*,[1] the Supreme Court
ruled that any evidentiary material taken in an unreasonable search
cannot be used against the person from whom it was improperly
obtained in any court of law. This is called the exclusionary rule of
evidence because such evidence is selectively excluded in a trial on the
merits of the case involving such information or physical evidence.

The history of cases related to search have established it is a
fundamental rule that a search without a warrant is not reasonable
unless an arrest is involved. If an individual is to be searched without

Probable cause: more than a suspicion, but less than a certainty that a
crime has been committed
Absolute right: complete, without any condition or incumberance
Qualified right: gives the possessor a right for certain purposes or under
certain circumstances only

[1]   *Mapp v. Ohio*, 367 U.S. 643 (1961).

a warrant, or without the individual consenting to the search, there must be an arrest. The general rule is that if the search precedes the arrest, and the search provides the basis or probable cause, the search would be *ipso facto*, an unreasonable search.

The courts recognize the police officers' right to seize instruments, contraband, and the fruits of crime that are in plain view. This is referred to as the plain view doctrine.

In the present case, one main issue is that the patients, Jesse and Jeffrey James, are not under arrest. If the patients were under arrest, Sergeant Hoover would be justified in searching the arrestees, their clothing and personal effects. These same articles could be subjected to laboratory examination.

A warrant must describe the person, place, and things to be searched or seized with a reasonable degree of specificity. Exception to the general rule of requiring a warrant prior to searching an individual is where there is exigent circumstances and a clear indication that evidence would be removed or destroyed. For example, if an individual is arrested during a car accident the arresting officer can search the individual and the immediate area, but not the trunk of the car.

The patients, of course, could give expressed consent to a search, effectively waiving their fundamental right of protection as guaranteed by the Fourth Amendment. This waiver would have to be completely voluntary and understood to be an intentional waiver of their constitutional right.

The Fourth Amendment does not protect abandoned property. But there is nothing abandoned in the present case. There is at law the theory of custodial safety. In a 1960 federal court case [2] it was held that the law does not require return of property which could be used by a prisoner to harm himself or others. This case involved the protection of a prisoner and a prisoner's property.

The conclusion to be drawn is that, as a general rule, the health practitioner does not have the authority, the right, or the responsibility to search the patient. However, as with all, there is the common sense exception. It may happen that while caring for a patient, it comes to the attention of the health care practitioner that the patient has a weapon, such as a knife or gun, or a large amount of drugs.

Contraband: anything that is against law or treaty; prohibited
Exigent: immediate

2   *Charles v. U.S.*, 278 F. 2d 386 (1960).

If reasonable health care practitioners would conclude from the known fact that the patient may harm others or himself with the weapon or drugs, then the health care practitioner has a duty to act to protect the patient and other potential victims. The health care practitioner must take such action as is commensurate with the imminent danger to the safety and well being of all persons involved. If the immediate danger calls for removal of the specific items then they should be promptly removed. If the danger is not imminent but potentially dangerous, then the appropriate authorities, such as the administration or legal authorities, such as police, should be notified.

It is often general hospital policy that a patient admitted through the emergency room either conscious or unconscious will have his wallet removed for identification and safe keeping. Other items of value such as rings, clothing, etc. will either be given to the family members, if present, or placed for safekeeping by hospital personnel.

The key issue is that this limited search is permissible in a medical emergency for the purpose of ascertaining identity. The primary role of the health care practitioner is to treat the patient and give medical care. The role is not to assist the police officers in their investigation nor to serve as an independent investigator himself. This is not to say they should inhibit, obstruct or delay appropriate legal authorities while they are doing their job. But overzealous health care practitioners have been known to step out of their roles and act inappropriately and without authority in emergency room situations. To search citizens not under arrest at the request of a police officer could place the health care practitioner in the position of violating a patient's constitutional rights, however well intentioned the practitioner, searching a patient's personal effects.

In the vignette presented the first issue to be addressed is the legal obligation of either Sarah Gampie, R.N. or Kris Kritical, M.D. to conform to the request of Sergeant Edgett Hoover. The law is clear that the primary function of health care personnel is the health care of the patient brought to an emergency room. Therefore, there is no legal obligation on either health care practitioner. The second issue is whether the blood alcohol or blood barbiturate would have been ordered independent of the police officer's request by Dr. Kritical. If

Arrest [3]: an arrest is the taking, seizing, or detaining of another 1) by touching or putting hands on him; 2) by any act that indicates an intention to take him into custody and subject him to the actual control of the person making the arrest; or 3) by the consent of the person to be arrested.

[3] Amer. Jur., 2d. ARREST SECTION 1 (1962).

the procedures are part of the diagnostic and therapeutic regimen it would not be considered violative of the patient's rights. If it is ordered to acquiesce in the investigative officers request, it could be considered violative of the patient's rights. In a District of Columbia [4] appeals case the court said that intrusion into the human body is a greater invasion of privacy than searching clothing and greater indignity than police entering a home.

The patient might well have a cause of action against the health care practitioner who would perform a procedure without the patient's permission and for a non-therapeutic purpose. Most states have legislation specifically enacted to cover taking blood samples from patients. For example, New York grants immunity from liability for health care practitioners who comply with the request of police to take blood samples. Kansas, Maryland and Pennsylvania require the permission of the patient. If it involves a motor vehicle accident, the patient may still refuse to have a blood test. The refusal, however, results in immediate suspension of the license to drive a motor vehicle.

Any health care practitioner working in an emergency room should be aware of the laws of the state governing such requests. If the health care practitioner is not aware, a request in writing should be made to the hospital attorney through appropriate channels for clarification and advice in these and similar situations to prevent legal risk.

GUIDELINES AND CLOSING COMMENTS

Everyone wants a foolproof answer to their problems. This is truer in the legal area where inappropriate answers can be costly in monetary assessment for damages. There are general guidelines that can be given to arrive at the appropriate legal answer to avert legal liability or risk. They can also be used to establish appropriate policy when a potential legal risk situation arises. The guidelines are not all inclusive. But the guidelines, plus a professional approach, plus common sense should result in solutions to the majority of problems encountered.

The first guideline is to establish the authority for the particular action. Does the authorization arise from a recent case in the jurisdiction that covers such action? Is it a result of legislative enactments or statutes? Does hospital policy, state licensing bodies, or accrediting agencies require or recommend such action? Are there joint resolutions

---

4 *U.S. v. Crowder,* 513 F 2d. APP. D.C. 1975.

of medical or nursing societies that allow such actions? Are there any other documents emanating internally or externally from the health care agency that approve the actions taken or to be taken either expressly or inherently?

The second guideline is to establish the real purpose of a particular action. Are the actions compatible with the objective of the health care agency? Are the actions in the best interest of patient care or are they for the convenience of certain groups? Are the actions attempting to do something indirectly that should be done directly? We must be aware that our purpose must stand up to the scrutiny of the public. To say it is in the patient's best interest may not be enough. We may be called upon to prove it with facts and evidence and not simply statements.

In some states where there is doubt about the legality of a particular procedure, it is possible to get an Attorney General's opinion prior to doing a particular action. Since the Attorney General is the official legal advisor to the state government, only state or municipal organizations can be served by the Attorney General. However, the State Board of Examiners frequently will request an Attorney General's opinion on a particular subject and promulgate the opinion to registered and licensed professionals.

A fourth consideration is to establish an ongoing joint practice, multidisciplinary committee. This committee would have access to all necessary data related to risk situations and proposed policy. The committee recommend training programs as needed on an ongoing basis. For example, where there has been a high incidence of medication errors, the committee could study the problem and make recommendations that certain personnel be required to take a prescribed course in pharmacy. The committee could make recommendations in other areas for proposed policy or policy revisions. The recommendations could be made directly to the administrator. These recommendations, if accepted, could become the basis for action by health care practitioners.

An area neglected by nurses is to request a legal opinion from the hospital attorney. He is the appropriate party from whom to request legal advice regarding any situations in which there is concern regarding legal liability. Although it may be proper procedurally to proceed through the supervisor or director of nurses, as far as protocol is concerned, no health care practitioner should flounder in ignorance regarding legal obligations. A good method when there are recurrent problems is to write the problem as succinctly and comprehensively as possible. Send the problem on to the hospital attorney according to proper channels and policy and request a written legal opinion or advice on the problem.

Finally, nurses should get in the habit of seeking consultation with another nurse. When faced with a difficult situation, discuss it with a peer. This does several things. It gives another presumably objective opinion. It helps establish the standard of care because in reality you are establishing what another reasonably prudent nurse would do in the same set of circumstances. As a result of this, you have a corroborating witness of the events that have taken place. If prudence dictates it, you and the consulting peer could document and record what the problem was, what action was taken and why, and sign and witness the record. This type of action could be very persuasive if any of the events led to litigation.

By following these guidelines you are not guaranteed victory in an adversary proceeding, but you are guaranteed to be a formidable opponent.

Guidelines to answer legal problems or establish policy to prevent legal problems:

1. By what authority.
2. For what purpose.
3. Attorney General's opinion or other legal official.
4. Joint practice, multidisciplinary committee.
5. Requesting legal opinions or advice from hospital attorney or health care agency's legal counsel.
6. Consultation with peer.

Conclusion

In conclusion, the authors would give the reader a final scintilla of advice. In talking with nurses across the nation, the question has been asked of these dedicated health professionals: who is the most important person in the hospital? The response to the question is unequivocally a loud resounding "the patient." The authors disagree with this answer. We submit to you that the most important person in the institution is "you." Remember the words *cui bono*, "for whose best interest." As the nurse, the authors would agree with the commitment that the patient is the most important person. As the attorney, the best advice you can receive is to look out for your own interest. This is not said in the sense that others are adversaries. Nor is it the end product of professional paranoia. The nurse must use prudence and protect her interests. She must be aware of the legal risks involved in the work situations, and take appropriate action to protect her interests. It is doubtful anyone else will do this for her. *Cui bono!*

Part Four
APPENDICES

APPENDIX I   HISTORY

The basic principles of American law and the prevailing legal philosophy is derived almost entirely from the English legal system. Western civilization has essentially two concepts of legal thought, the English, or *common law* system and the European, or *civil law* system. The *civil law* system was developed from Roman law. Civil law is a "civil code" system adopted by the legislature. It is fundamentally a collection of basic principles to be applied to individual cases. Louisiana is the only state which retains a modified civil law resulting from its French heritage.

Civil law approach to the solution of legal problems may be compared to the concept of deductive reasoning. Preestablished general principles are applied to individual cases.

Common law is a system of inductive reasoning where the general principle is derived from an accumulation of decisions in particular cases.

In early England, the King appointed judges to travel the country and settle differences and disputes among the population. It became evident that similar fact situations should be decided in the same way by the judges to establish consistency. This would enable an individual to reasonably predict the legal consequences of his behavior. This concept became *precedent*; that is, in the absence of any other guide to a decision, a court will follow a previous decision on the same subject made by another court.

In today's complex court hierarchy, the doctrine means a lower court must follow the decisions of a higher court in its jurisdiction, even if the judge disagrees with that decision. A trial court in any state is required to follow the precedents established by the appellate courts of that state and all state courts must follow the rulings of the Supreme Court of the United States.

Where there is no precedent established by a higher court, courts of equal rank generally tend, but are not required, to follow the decisions of sister states.

APPENDIX II   CLASSIFICATIONS OF LAW AFFECTING HEALTH CARE PROFESSIONALS

The law affects the health care professional in many aspects of his working life. Are you aware of what kinds of law affect you while working in health care centers? When asked this question, most health care practitioners respond with malpractice law as the answer. This is probably because today most of us are concerned with lawsuits; however, we are affected by other classifications of law.

Contract Law   Contract law plays a significant part in our everyday lives. We make contracts with our employers, our patients, and our co-workers. Granted, it may be a very informal proceeding; nevertheless the elements of a contract are often present. Contract law is a subcategory of civil law. Professional relationships with patients are often based on implied understanding rather than expressed written agreements.

Criminal Law   Criminal law is an area most health care practitioners are aware of as it relates to narcotics, assault and battery, and in some cases, abortions. How many health care practitioners are aware that doing certain actions could be construed as practicing medicine and that these actions would be illegal? For example, it is not unusual for a nurse to decide to reduce a particular medication, such as demerol from 100 mg. to 50 mg., because the nurse believes a lesser amount is appropriate in a particular case. Or, if a patient is in pain, a nurse may give an analgesic previously ordered by a doctor when the nurse cannot locate the doctor. Although intentions in both

Malpractice: negligent or improper conduct of professional persons
Assault: threat to do bodily harm
Battery: committing bodily harm

examples are commendable, both are illegal acts and the nurse would be practicing medicine without a license.

Constitutional Law   Today we are more aware of human rights, both the patients' rights and the health practitioners' rights. The law governing rights is generally classified as *constitutional law* and it is becoming more important each day in the health care field. No longer can a health care agency treat patients as second class citizens. Patients remain citizens protected by the U.S. Constitution even though they enter health care agencies or institutions. No rights are waived simply because an individual becomes a patient. Also, the health care institution cannot negate any of the patients' rights under the guise of "doing what is best for the patient." The patient is expected to be the main participant and decision-maker in his health care.

Administrative Law   Never before have we been so inundated by rules and regulations from outside agencies. The federal government and state governments are assuming more and more responsibility for health care. Accreditation and licensing bodies, federal and state governments, and medicare dictate directly or indirectly many of the policies, procedures, and functions of health care institutions. This comes under the classification of *administrative law*. Administrative law is a specialized area of law. A specific governmental agency of either the federal government or the state government is charged with administering particular legislation. Some examples of administrative agencies are the state health department, state board of medical examiners, and the state board of nurse examiners.

For those institutions that provide a grievance procedure, this would also come under administrative law. The law states that one must "exhaust his administrative remedies" before one can go to court. This means that where an institution has provided a grievance procedure as an internal method for remedying disagreements, it must be followed. In administrative law actions, it is important to adhere to the procedural specifications as well as the substantive specifications. Where a procedure states a petition must be filled in a certain way or an answer must be given in a certain number of days, it must be done as mandated. It is essential to be careful, because if you do not follow administrative procedure, you could inadvertently waive your

Constitutional Law: branch of law dealing with organization and function of government

Administrative Law: branch of law dealing with organs of government power and prescribes in detail the manner of their activity

rights. You could lose your case because you failed to follow prescribed procedure and never get to the merits of the issues.

Labor Relations Law A knowledge of the labor relations law is essential as more and more health care workers become unionized. It is necessary to know what is acceptable legal activity for management and for employees. Health care practitioners could be participating in unfair labor practices and not be aware of it because of inexperience and lack of knowledge. Lack of experience or lack of knowledge or both would not excuse such activity in the eyes of the law, and individuals could be held liable for illegal union activity.

Uniform Commercial Code Few health care practitioners view the Uniform Commercial Code as having any impact on their professional lives. Yet in our advanced technological age the need to understand warranties and preconditions to action, for breach of warranty, is unprecedented. The manufacturer of hospital equipment generally warrants the equipment to be fit for its intended purpose and free from defect. The hospital staff must comply with the stipulations made in the manufacturer's warranty to keep the warranty in effect. Improvisation was a commendable attribute in an employee years ago and one often advocated by instructors in the health care field. Today with the complexity of technology, one should improvise, if at all, with prudent reflection. Instructions for equipment should be read and followed. Classes should be held to teach the use of new equipment so all employees understand the function and the warranty involved in the use of the equipment.

Medical Malpractice Law The medical malpractice law affects health care workers daily as they are charged with treating every patient with "due care," and acting as a reasonably prudent professional person in the particular circumstances.

All these different classifications of law—civil, criminal, constitutional, administrative and commercial medical malpractice—are implemented in the health care structure. The affect and effect of law on the professional life of a health care practitioner is more comprehensive than simply that of medical negligence. The law is a behavioral–political–sociological oriented discipline. As health care situations are analyzed, the relationship between the above classifications of law and one's health care activity are more easily recognized. It is acknowledgedly beyond the scope of this text to analyze each classification of law in detail. But this is an attempt to alert the reader that there is more involved in rules of conduct relating to one's profession than malpractice law.

APPENDIX III   COURT SYSTEM

Review of Court System

A brief review of the court system is presented to give you an appreciation of the procedural aspects necessary to move a care to its ultimate resolution. A *court* is the forum where justice is administered. The judge and jury serve as neutral arbitrators of the facts and evidence presented to them.

Courts are generally classed as either *lower* or *superior courts.* The term lower or *inferior court* implies that the court has limited authority. Usually each state sets out in its statutes the types of cases a court will hear and the maximum money value of the cases over which it will have jurisdiction.

The United States Constitution, formally adopted in 1789, created our legal system. Essentially there are two systems: 1) the federal and 2) the state or local system. The founders of the Constitution were very purposeful in creating this system. Their main purpose was to prevent a monarchy, or a monopoly of power. This is a basic concept of our system of government. It is a system of checks and balances to prevent too much power in the hands of one branch of government.

Federal Judicial System

The federal judicial system has at least one United States district court in each of the states depending on the population of the state. These courts are courts of general jurisdiction having power to determine cases involving a citizen's personal civil rights or criminal acts involving federal laws. There are certain cases that only a federal court may hear and therefore the federal court is said to have *exclusive* jurisdiction over particular types of cases, for example, maritime or copyright matters. The Constitution or Congress has authorized these federal courts only to hear such cases. Such courts would be in the U.S. Court of Claims which hears cases or claims against the United States government, or the Tax Court of the United States which hears cases involving federal tax matters.

The courts of appeals for both the United States district courts and the United States courts of limited or exclusive jusisdiction are the United States Courts of Appeals, also called *circuit courts,* because of the geographical region or circuit into which they are divided.

The final court of appeal in the federal system is the United States Supreme Court. A decision made by this highest appellate court becomes the "law of the land" for all citizens of the United States. (See Exhibit 3.)

FEDERAL COURT SYSTEM

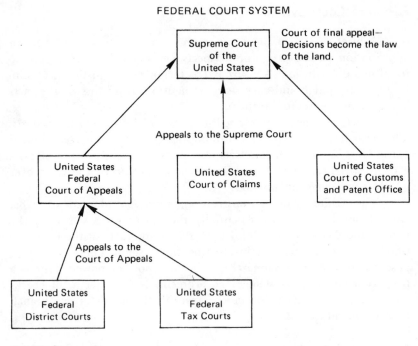

Exhibit 3.

These courts could be limited regarding the amount of money involved, for example, only hearing cases where damages are up to $5000. Amounts over this go into higher court. At the same time, they can have exclusive jurisdiction over certain subject matter, for example, automobile accidents involving citizens of two different states.

State and Local Judicial System

Essentially, the pattern and organization of the state courts is analogous to the federal judicial system. That is, there are inferior or lower courts of limited jurisdiction. Generally, there are specialized

Jurisdiction: the court has the authority to hear the case
Appellate: process to appeal a decision

courts such as family, traffic, probate or small claims courts. There is generally a comparable system to the federal courts of the lower trial court where a case is initially heard and the jury or judge determines the facts of a particular case. The judge then applies the law to the jury's finding. Where an individual has waived his right to a jury trial, the judge determines the facts.

The state then has a system of appeal where an individual can request a higher court (appellate court) to review the lower court's decision. This is considered an intermediate court of appeals. There is a final court of appeal in each state to the state Supreme Court (sometimes called Court of Appeals of the state) and the decisions of that particular court are the law of the particular state. Where there is a constitutional question involved in any state case, the appellant may appeal to the United States Supreme Court. (See Exhibit 4.)

Scope of Jurisdiction and Appeal   There are three types of superior courts or appellate courts. They are: 1) United States District Courts, 2) State Superior Courts, and 3) Federal and State Appeals Courts. The United States District Courts have jurisdiction over bankruptcy cases, banking, maritime laws, federal crimes, federal civil actions, questions of constitutionality, violation of federal laws and treaties. They also decide controversies between citizens of different states and between two states or a state and the United States. At one time, an individual or group of individuals desiring to bring action against the government for a tort resulting in personal injury first had to obtain permission of the Congress to institute such action. This procedure was tedious, expensive, and slow. Now the United States Court of Claims has been established to expedite arbitration of these matters. A patient in a federally-managed hospital, for instance, who claims a personal injury from mismanagement of a medical problem appeals to the United States Court of Claims for redress.

Each state's courts are referred to as *lower* courts because the decisions of that court may be appealed to a *higher* court, known as the Court of Appeals, or the Supreme Court of the state. The terminology depends on the state. Generally, appeals courts consist of three to six judges who review the record of the proceedings in the lower court, the transcript, and the evidence on which the decision was based. They may remand the case, or they may overrule the lower court, i.e.,

Probate: proving wills or handling estates
Waive: renounce or give up a privilege
Appellant: one taking an appeal
Remand: send back

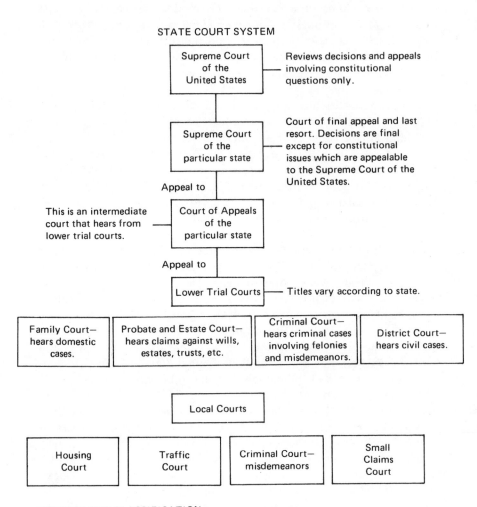

STATE COURT SYSTEM

Supreme Court
of the
United States

Reviews decisions and appeals involving constitutional questions only.

Supreme Court
of the
particular state

Court of final appeal and last resort. Decisions are final except for constitutional issues which are appealable to the Supreme Court of the United States.

Appeal to

This is an intermediate court that hears from lower trial courts.

Court of Appeals
of the
particular state

Appeal to

Lower Trial Courts — Titles vary according to state.

Family Court—
hears domestic
cases.

Probate and Estate Court—
hears claims against wills,
estates, trusts, etc.

Criminal Court—
hears criminal cases
involving felonies
and misdemeanors.

District Court—
hears civil cases.

Local Courts

Housing
Court

Traffic
Court

Criminal Court—
misdemeanors

Small
Claims
Court

DIVISION AND CLASSIFICATION

OF LOCAL AND LOWER TRIAL COURTS   Titles vary from state to state.

Exhibit 4.

the court of original jurisdiction where the decision was made, if the original judge has made a legal error, and remand the case for retrial.

Each state has a court system which permits the decisions of each court to be reviewed or appealed to a higher court within the state. These courts are referred to as lower courts. Similarly, the federal judicial system has circuit courts of appeals composed of judges who review lower court decisions.

An appeal may be made from the various lower courts in a state to the final Court of Appeals or Supreme Court of the state. (Court of Appeals and Supreme Court are synonymous terms depending on the state). These state Supreme Courts are composed of five to nine judges who review the decisions of the lower or intermediate court of appeals. The review of the decision is to see if the lower court judge was arbitrary or capricious or if the law was improperly applied.

Lower Trial and Appeal Procedure   The trial in the lower courts involves the admission of testimony of witnesses, viewing of records, and examination of actual objects or exhibits involved in committing the crime or wrong against society or an individual. The lower court trial may take hours or weeks depending on the type and amount of evidence introduced. The *plaintiff* or accuser and the *defendant* or the accused are present in the courtroom throughout the entire proceedings. In the appeals process the plaintiff and the defendant do not appear in the appellate court; instead, their attorneys present arguments for or against the verdict or ruling of the original presiding judge. Following this, the court of appeals either upholds the verdict of the lower court, reverses the decision, or orders a retrial if the judge erred in a matter of law during the trial.

The criminal trial is an interesting one to follow as an example of court procedure. Here legal arguments and technicalities are extremely important because the defendant's freedom hangs in the balance. At the opening of trial, the bailiff or judge announces to the court the criminal charges against the defendant. At this time, the defendant is asked whether he wants to be tried before the judge at the district court level, or whether he wants a trial by jury as a constitutional right. The defendant elects (chooses) if the case is to be tried by the judge or jury, and the trial begins. During the trial, the defense attorney must make timely motion, such as the suppression of evidence, legality of the arrest, the sequestering of witness, and various other technical defenses that may be applicable. The attorney must raise these issues and defenses at the beginning of the trial; then the case is tried on the merits of the facts presented.

First, the state presents its case by putting its witnesses on the stand; afterwards, the defense may cross-examine these witnesses. At the end of the state's case, the defense counsel makes a timely motion for verdict of acquittal based on legal argument. The court, after listening to the argument, will either sustain or deny the motion for

Defendant: person being sued or prosecuted
Plaintiff: person suing or bringing the action

verdict of acquittal. In the event that the defense counsel's motions are denied, he must go forward with the defense for his client.

At this time, the defense counsel (in open court) informs his client again of his constitutional right to remain silent and that there is no inference of guilt should he remain silent. The defense counsel then informs the court of his client's wish, and the defense begins. The defense counsel proceeds by calling witnesses, if any, on behalf of the defense. After the conclusion of all testimony by the defense and all cross-examination by the state, the defense then renews his motions for acquittal, arguing both the facts and the law. The state then rebuts. If the court fails to grant the motions of the defense, the jury retires to a room to discuss the evidence and decide if the defendant is guilty or innocent of the charges. The judge then announces the verdict.

If a guilty verdict is reached by the jury, the court gives the defense an opportunity to argue in *mitigation* on behalf of his client, initially trying to secure probation, or failing this, trying to secure a minimal or lenient sentence for his client. The argument in mitigation is based on the fact that there were extenuating circumstances to cause the defendant to act as he did. Another argument might be that the plaintiff's actions were such that they do not justify the defendant being punished so severely. The judge then imposes the sentence.

At the end of the trial, the judge informs the defendant of his rights of appeal.

This presentation of court proceedings is to demonstrate the orderly process the courts implement to assure due process and a fair hearing to all citizens. It is a simple analysis of the federal and state court system to be used as a tool in understanding the comprehensiveness of the legal system.

APPENDIX IV   AUTHORITY

Authority Determines Liability

Authority, according to Black's Law Dictionary, is the legal power or the right to act or command. The authority for the health

Sequestering: isolating
Verdict of acquittal: argument that there is not sufficient evidence against the defendant to proceed and case should be dismissed
Mitigation: allievation; abatement or diminution of a penalty imposed by law

care center is derived from its charter. The charter establishes the board of trustees as the ultimate legal authority in the corporation. All other authority, including the hospital administration, who is sometimes referred to as the chief executive officer, and the medical staff or the nursing administration, is delegable authority.

Authority, or legal power, is the basis for determining responsibility, accountability, and liability. Any realistic analysis of authority soon establishes that it is the most fundamental concept in law or in organizational development. One must be concerned with authority to set in perspective the related aspects of theories of liability and responsibility. The subject of authority must be recognized as the essential ingredient underlying an understanding of the roles and relationships in the health field. The first consideration in ascertaining function, roles, and responsibilities is to ask the question, "By what authority?". The answer to this seemingly innocuous question often will indicate within what professional and legal scope we are safely functioning.

Creation of Authority

How does a hospital or health care center come into being? How does a hospital or health care center assume authority and responsibility for health care of certain citizenry? The institution generally incorporates. The authority of a governing board of an institution arises from the statutory laws of the state regarding incorporation. The existence of this authority inherently creates duties, obligations, and liabilities. The basic document creating the corporation is the charter. The charter is granted to a specific institution through the Secretary of State of the particular jurisdiction through the articles of incorporation. Because it is created by law the corporation possesses only the authority and power conferred on it in the charter. The charter in turn confers upon the governing body of the corporation the right to enact bylaws, policies, and procedures for establishing the orderly operation of the health care center.

The charter of the corporation establishes the nature and purpose of the corporation. Generally, the charter will state the expressed powers of the corporation and imply that there is inherent power to perform those expressed without detailing the implied power. When a governing body, such as a board of directors or trustees, enacts and adopts bylaws to regulate the functioning of the health care center, those bylaws have the force of law for the health care center. They are in effect the bill of rights for the corporation or health care center. Who has the authority in a health care setting? The language of recent judicial decisions removes all doubt as to who has the authority and the responsibility for patient care. The first-line responsibility is the board of trustees.

The traditional role of health care providers is being reinterpreted and new legal relationships are being defined. The governing body of the hospital or health center is the board of trustees. Case law, statutes, and standards of accreditation all recognize the ultimate, nondelegable corporate and legal responsibility of the board to assure that quality care is provided. Vesting of the legal responsibility for patient care is more clearly recognized and understood today than ever before. Each judicial decision reaffirms the fact that the governing boards of health centers have the ultimate responsibility for the operation and function of the agency and for providing proper patient care.

The board is charged with the right and the duty to monitor the quality of health care being provided by the professional staff. It has the final authority to satisfy the corporate objectives. All others, administrator, medical staff and nursing staff, have delegated authority to act within defined parameters of operations. The actual monitoring of the quality of health care being delivered should be delegated to the medical and nursing staff because they, by professional training and experience, are most capable of performing this important task.

Institutional Authority Guidelines   All health care practitioners should be knowledgeable about the policies and procedures of the institution in which they are employed. Policies are developed in accordance wtih the health care agencies' objectives. Policies are guidelines within which employees of an institution must operate and make appropriate decisions compatible with those policies.

Procedures are a series of steps outlined by the institution or health care agency to accomplish a specific objective or task. For example, a grievance procedure is highly structured and must be followed step by step to develop into a "fair hearing," the ultimate objective. There are procedures for transfusing blood, obtaining narcotics, and requesting time off. Procedures are necessary to an institution to give orderly uniformity to certain routine functions.

Rules and regulations are generally clear and concise statements mandating or prohibiting certain activity in the institution. A hospital rule or regulation might dictate what type of attire is to be worn in certain units such as the operating room, nursery, intensive care unit

Case law: decisions by the courts
Statute: legislative enactments
Standards: criteria of measuring

and other special areas. Similarly, a health care agency might prohibit all smoking in patient care areas.

A job description is written in broad terms and this document is part of the composite documents to determine by what authority action is taken. For example, a job description would describe a supervisor's authority over certain areas such as the Intensive Care Unit or the Coronary Care Unit. This would imply that the supervisor has inherent authority to carry out those job functions. There is implicit authority to do the job competently although every specific act is not spelled out. There is usually a catch-all phrase at the end of the nurse's job description that says something comparable to "and whatever else the Director of Nurses in her discretion deems necessary." Nurses sometimes interpret this to mean the Director of Nurses can tell them to do anything and they must comply. This is not true. The term, as always, means what is reasonable to expect a particular individual of the same academic qualifications and training to be able to accomplish. The Director of Nurses would be acting inappropriately were she to assign a recent nursing graduate to take charge of duties in the Intensive Care Unit without appropriate training and orientation. The Director of Nurses could not point to the broad terms of a job description and say that this clause gives her authority to send this nurse to any unit at any time. This would be construed as an unreasonable interpretation and probably negligent action.

External Influences   There are various internal and external forces which dictate the health care practice. Examples of these include state licensing agencies for individuals, as well as institutions, state board of examiners' rules and regulations, accreditation agencies, federal regulations—medicare and medicaid, agencies to enforce occupational health and safety acts, labor unions and their contracts, Blue Cross and Blue Shield regulations, professional staff review organizations, medical audit—internal and external, and quality assurance reviews—internal and external.

These are listed simply to impress that authority to do general or specific acts can result from expressed and implied authority or from internal or external sources. They also present the fact that authorization is necessary in some form to function as health care practitioners or legal risk may be imminent.

These agencies, processes, mechanisms and other mandates prohibit, influence, or affect the health care practitioner's activity.

Nevertheless, the relationship of authority to one's function and responsibilities and its importance to legal liability can be better understood by an awareness of the internal and external factors that are determinative.

Part Five

EVALUATION OF PROCESSED CONTENT

SECTION A   DEFINITIONS

DEFINE THE FOLLOWING DOCTRINES AND PRINCIPLES OF LAW FREQUENTLY APPLIED IN LITIGATION INVOLVING HEALTH CARE.

1. Rule of Personal Liability
2. Corporate Negligence
3. Respondeat Superior
4. Borrowed Servant Doctrine
5. Reasonably Prudent Man Doctrine
6. Foreseeability
7. Res Ipsa Loquitur
8. Statute of Limitations
9. Contributory Negligence
10. Comparative Negligence
11. Outrageous Conduct

SECTION B   TRUE/FALSE ITEMS

The following items may be viewed as a possible multiple choice in which the response options are limited to either a true or a false selection.

The task is to determine which statement is true or false by marking *T* for a true statement or *F* for a false statement.

1. *Common law* and *judicial decisions* are terms that can be used interchangeably.
2. *Statutory law* and *legislative enactments* are terms that can be used interchangeably.
3. *Common law* and *legislative enactments* are synonymous terms.
4. An example of a judicial decision is the court opinion in the *Darling v. Charleston Community Hospital* case defining the doctrine of corporate negligence.
5. An example of statutory law is the Nurse Practice Act.
6. An act committed by a health care practitioner involving assault and battery on a patient must be either a *Tort* or a *Crime*. It cannot meet both definitions simultaneously.
7. Criminal law deals with conduct which offends society as a whole and not just the individual victim of the crime.
8. Statutory law deals with conduct which offends one or more individuals in society.
9. A health care practitioner who fails to act reasonably and prudently is considered to be negligent in the eyes of the law.
10. Malpractice refers to the negligence of a professional person who has failed to meet the standard of care of professional persons.
11. The law of negligence is a sub-classification of the Law of Malpractice.
12. The legal doctrine of respondeat superior applies to the acts of medical personnel only.
13. The doctrine of corporate negligence states that the corporation has failed to follow established standards of conduct to which it is expected to conform.
14. The doctrine of foreseeability holds that governments and municipalities cannot be held liable for their employees.
15. Statutory law is distinguished from judicial decisions in that statutory law is derived from the ethics of common law.
16. Generally, patients are expected to act as reasonably, prudent patients only under certain circumstances.
17. The branch of law which deals with mutual agreements and patient injuries is criminal law.
18. A competent adult patient has the right to refuse medication or treatment at any time.
19. It is unnecessary to obtain an informed consent from an unconscious patient brought to the emergency room because the law presumes the patient wants to be treated.

20. A nurse who acts carefully and prudently will not be deemed negligent for any of her professional nursing activities.

SECTION C   MULTIPLE CHOICE ITEMS

Select one response from the options given which you believe to be the correct or best answer available.

1. The branch of law which deals with mutual agreements and understanding is part of:

a. Contract law
b. Constitutional law
c. Criminal law
d. Commercial law
e. Tort law

2. The branch of law which deals with conduct that is less than reasonable under the particular circumstances is a part of:

a. Contract law
b. Constitutional law
c. Criminal law
d. Commercial law
e. Tort law

2. The branch of law which deals with the inherent rights of patients is part of:

a. Contract law
b. Constitutional law
c. Labor-Relations law
d. Commercial law
e. Tort law

4. The branch of law which deals with the inherent rights of health care practitioners is a part of:

a. Contract law
b. Constitutional law
c. Labor-Relations law

d. Commercial law
e. Tort law

5. The branch of law which deals with implied and expressed warranties is a part of:

a. Contract law
b. Constitutional law
c. Criminal law
d. Commercial law

6. The branch of law which deals with conduct that is offensive to society as a whole and against the public interest is a part of:

a. Contract law
b. Constitutional law
c. Criminal law
d. Commercial law

7. An example of a contractual arrangement between a health care practitioner and a patient is which of the following:

a. The health care practitioner provides health care to the patient
b. There is a verbal agreement between the health care practitioner and the patient
c. There is a written agreement between the health care practitioner and the patient
d. All of the above

8. A patient who fails to act in a reasonably prudent manner and is injured as a result may be considered to be:

a. Medically negligent
b. Contributorily negligent
c. Immune due to status as a patient
d. None of the above

9. If an individual is found to be negligent in a civil case, what are the expected consequences as a result of a verdict of negligence?

a. Individual will be expected to pay a fine or serve a jail term
b. Individual will be expected to pay assessed money damages

   c. Individual will be required to have a hearing before appropriate board of professional examiners

   d. Individual will automatically forfeit his license

10. If an individual is found guilty in a criminal case the defendant:

   a. will automatically forfeit his license

   b. will be expected to pay assessed money damages

   c. will be expected to pay a fine or serve a jail term

   d. All of the above

11. A health care practitioner:

   a. always has the right to question a physician's order.

   b. never has the right to question a physician's order

   c. must meet certain criteria before questioning a physician's order

   d. none of the above

12. Restraints may be applied against a patient's will in certain circumstances, such as:

   a. on a physician's order

   b. a patient is injurious to himself or other patients

   c. shortage of staff

   d. the family has requested it

13. Restraining a patient without consent, proper authorization, or specific criteria could result in an allegation against the health care practitioner of:

   a. assault and battery.

   b. legal irresponsibility.

   c. breach of contract.

   d. malpractice.

14. A health care practitioner who fails to act in a reasonably prudent manner when performing acts of a professional nature may be charged with:

   a. Tortious action

   b. Negligence

c. Malpractice
d. Gross negligence

15. Consent to operate forms should be signed by a patient:

a. after a complete explanation of the procedure by the nurse.
b. after a complete explanation of the risks involved by the physician.
c. in the presence of two witnesses.
d. All of the above.

16. An incident report form should be completed:

a. for any untoward accident involving a patient.
b. for every medication error.
c. immediately and a copy placed on patient's chart.
d. immediately and a copy sent to the hospital attorney.
e. according to the agency's policy.

17. Medical records and charts are important and necessary documents for which of the following:

a. Communication between health care practitioners and agencies
b. Legal evidence as documentation of certain patient events
c. Research and statistical information for various governmental agencies.
d. Medical audits and accreditation and licensing process
e. All of the above

18. Medical records and charts keeping should be:

a. specific, concise, accurate, irrelevant.
b. factual rather than opinionated.
c. source oriented rather than problem oriented.
d. recognized as diminishing in value in the age of computers.

19. A legal signature on a document such as a medical record should have:

a. name only.
b. name plus professional status.

c. sufficient data to assure specific identification.

d. variations according to shift and agency policy.

20. An unconscious patient is brought into the emergency unit bleeding profusely. The informed consent should:

a. be held unnecessary under the circumstances.

b. be signed by the next-to-kin, i.e., parent, spouse, child.

c. be signed by the hospital administrator under agency policy.

d. be signed by the patient as soon as condition warrants it.

SECTION D   SITUATIONS

Briefly discuss the legal risks and describe the legal implications to be considered in each of the following situations. The suggested answers are found in the previously presented vignettes as indicated by the numbers.

1. Patient John Doe was transferred from the City Hospital to a state operated nursing home. The staff at the nursing home observed that John Doe had a tendency to wander and act like a three-year-old child, going into temper tantrums when restricted in any way. The head nurse tried to contact the Nursing Administration at the City Hospital to get the history and certain medical data relevant to John Doe. The head nurse believed this information would assist them in planning proper patient care for Mr. John Doe. The Nursing Service Administrator declined to give any information on the basis it would be an invasion of John Doe's privacy and she had no authority to forward the medical records. She also stated all the information was on computer and automated data process and therefore required an even higher degree of confidentiality. *What, if any, are some legal risks involved?*

     Answer   Vignette 1

2. A patient on one of your psychiatric units refuses to take his medication because he feels that the medication will kill him. The patient's physician writes an order stating that the patient must have the medication; any route of administration is permissible—that is, oral, intramuscu-

lar, as long as the patient gets the medicine. You inform the physician that the patient refuses to take the medicine. In turn, he says that the patient must have the medicine. *What, if any, are some legal risks involved?*

Answer   Vignette 2

3. You are the only Registered Nurse on a geriatric ward with 30 to 35 patients. You are in charge of the 3 to 11 shift. Every morning, two or three patients who are quite elderly get active, at times even combative. You are concerned that these patients will hurt themselves or other patients. The private physicians refuse to write restraining orders because the patients are always quiet when the doctor sees them. The Evening Supervisor has told you to restrain these patients when you believe it necessary and she will support you if there is any problem. *What, if any, are some legal risks involved?*

Answer   Vignette 3

4. You are the Charge Nurse on a floor with thirty-five patients. Students of nursing from a nearby community college affiliate with your hospital. Each day you have on your unit three or four different students. Every day after the students leave you find patients assigned to students who have not been completely cared for; that is, baths not complete, procedures not done. You have been told by Nursing Administration that you are responsible for all the patients. You have also been told that the affiliating instructor is totally responsible for the students and you are not to interfere with the students. *What, if any, are some legal risks involved?*

Answer   Vignette 4

5. A new policy has been introduced at your hospital. Registered Nurses are to countersign for all nursing entries in patients' charts and for all medications given by nursing staff who are not Licensed Nurses. This policy includes Licensed Practical Nurses, and Nursing Students if the instructor is not present. If the instructor is

present, she is to countersign all the nursing care given by students. *What, if any, are some legal risks involved?*

Answer   Vignette 5

6. You are preparing Mrs. Smith for a hysterectomy operation and are about to have her sign the consent form. She signs the form and says, "My doctor hasn't discussed this surgery with me, but I guess he will before he operates, won't he?" *What, if any, are some legal risks involved?*

Answer   Vignette 6 & 7

7. Dr. Willis consistently writes orders that are very difficult to read. On this particular morning he writes a medication order without a clear indication of the administration route. *What, if any, are some legal risks involved?*

Answer   Vignette 8

8. The patient has an order for demerol, 100 mg. She is a patient who is three days post-operative for an appendectomy. The patient complains of "some pain—not too bad." You know it is customary to "split medications" on your floor. However, you are not sure about your authority in deciding to give 50 mg. now and 50 mg. later. *What, if any, are some legal risks involved?*

Answer   Vignette 16

9. You are the Supervisor on evening duty in a 300-bed hospital and receive a call from the nurse on duty in the emergency room. She states that a patient who was in an automobile accident and has a fractured femur is attempting to leave the hospital against medical advice. *What, if any, are some legal risks involved?*

Answer   Vignette 9

10. The work schedules are posted at least two months in advance. One particular evening a technician was scheduled to work 4 to 12 P.M. He did not come to work nor did he call. This has happened once before. The follow-

ing evening he comes to work when he is scheduled to be off. As the nurse in charge, you ask the technician where he had been the previous evening. He says that he forgot that he was supposed to work and came to work this evening to make up the time. *What, if any, are some legal risks involved?*

Answer   Vignette 10

11. You are a Staff Nurse on duty in the emergency room. You have been observing poor and inadequate care being given in the emergency room by physicians over a period of months. On two occasions you reported verbally two untoward incidents that took place in the emergency room to the Director of Nurses regarding similar incidents that involved poor patient care. Nothing happened. You have reason to believe you would not have administrative support if you continue reporting to the Director of Nurses. *What, if any, are some legal risks involved?*

Answer   Vignette 11

12. You are riding in the elevator with one of your colleagues; she begins to give a detailed account of a patient's condition, and you feel uncomfortable about continuing the discussion. Furthermore, you suspect that some of the patient's relatives are standing a few persons away from you. *What, if any, are some legal risks involved?*

Answer   Vignette 12

13. You are a nurse in the Coronary Care Unit of a general acute hospital. Mr. Jones is a 68-year-old male in congestive heart failure. His private physician tells you not to resuscitate Mr. Jones if he should stop breathing but refuses to write the order. Around 11:30 P.M. Mr. Jones stops breathing. You are alone in Cardiac Unit. *What, if any, are some legal risks involved?*

Answer   Vignette 13

14. You are a nurse on the Oncology Unit of a General Hospital. Mrs. Smith is a 38-year-old terminal cancer patient. Her private physician tells you not to resuscitate Mrs. Smith if she stops breathing. When you ask him to write the order, he refuses to do so. Around 11:00 P.M. Mrs. Smith stops breathing. You are alone on the Oncology Unit. *What, if any, are some legal risks involved?*

Answer   Vignette 14

15. Mrs. Smith is being examined for possible vaginal infection. The resident doctor who is doing the examination calls in three medical students to observe. *What, if any, are some legal risks involved?*

Answer   Vignette 15

16. Defective Equipment
You are working in the Clinical area. On evening report the Head Nurse tells you the suction equipment is "acting funny." She further states and demonstrates at the same time that she pressed the tube in two or three places to get it to work and you could do the same on your shift until the defective equipment could be fixed in the morning. There are two patients with the order "Suction P.R.N." What, if any, are your legal responsibilities? *What, if any, are some legal risks involved?*

Answer   Vignette 16

17. While making rounds, a Supervisor observed an elderly semi-comatose patient shivering and cold. The Supervisor directed the Head Nurse (a registered nurse) to apply hot water bottles to the patient. It was later discovered the patient had suffered first degree burns on both legs. *What, if any, are some legal risks involved?* Who, if anyone, would be held liable? What principles would apply?

Answer   Vignette 19

18. An elderly 72-year-old patient is having difficulty in breathing because of fluid in the lung. The doctor orders a thoracentesis stat. The patient requests her daughter be contacted before the procedure begins. You try in vain to contact the daughter as requested. The patient becomes progressively worse.
Can the doctor proceed with the thoracentesis?
What, if any, will be the liabilities should the thoracentesis be done?
Who, if anyone, will be liable?
What are some of the legal issues involved?

Answer   Vignette 6 & 7

19. Nurse White, R.N., is the Primary Care Nurse for John Black—a terminal cancer patient. Mr. Black complains of severe pain in his chest. Nurse White calls Dr. Jones, and describes the situation. Dr. Jones orders 75 mg. of demerol I.M. Nurse White administers it. Four hours later John Black again complains of severe chest pain. Nurse White tries in vain to contact Dr. Jones. The patient is becoming progressively more uncomfortable. After trying to get Dr. Jones in vain for over an hour, Nurse White repeats the 75 mg. of demerol I.M. again. The patient relaxes and rests comfortably; relieved from pain and no harm results.
Would there be any liability in this situation?
Who, if anyone, could be liable?
What is the legal basis for saying the health care practitioner would be liable?
What is the legal basis for saying the health care practitioner would not be liable?

Answer   Vignette 16

20. You are a Staff Nurse in the Emergency Room. Risk Management Data indicate the Emergency Room is an area of high legal liability. You are concerned about your malpractice liability coverage. In discussing this issue with your Supervisor, she states, "There is no need to worry—we have been told that all the Nursing Staff are covered by the hospital's insurance." *What, if any, are some legal risks involved?*

Answer   Vignette 25

ANSWERS

Section A   Answers to Definitions:

1. Rule of Personal Liability   A fundamental rule of law which holds that every person is liable for his own tortious conduct. The individual who is negligent is personally liable even though others are also liable.

2. Corporate Negligence   This means that the hospital as an entity is negligent. It is the failure of those entrusted with the task of providing the accommodations and facilities to carry out the purpose of the corporation and the failure to follow in a given situation the established standards of conduct to which the corporation should conform.

3. Doctrine of Respondeat Superior   "Let the master respond." This doctrine holds the employer legally responsible for the negligent acts of the employee. Two conditions must exist. One, there must be an employer-employee relationship and two, the employee must be functioning within the scope of his authority.

4. Borrowed Servant Doctrine   Theoretically, the hospital employs the individual but "loans" the individual to physician or agency. Any acts of negligence on the employee's part becomes the responsibility of the individual physician or agency to whom the employee was loaned. The controlling party is generally held liable for the acts of the employee over whom he had control.

5. Reasonably Prudent Man Doctrine   The standard of conduct expected to be used by an individual in an actual situation and represents the community ideal of the reasonable actions which a man of ordinary prudence would exercise in a hypothetical set of similar circumstances. It is difficult to establish definite rules because everything is relative to the particular situation.

6. Doctrine of Foreseeability   If an individual acts negligently towards another to whom a duty is owed to use due care, he is liable for all the natural and proximate consequences which could or should have been reasonably foreseen by the individual.

7. Doctrine of Res Ipsa Loquitur   "The thing speaks for itself." This doctrine raises a presumption of the defendant's negligence, but this presumption is a rebuttable one. Certain elements must be established before this doctrine can be utilized; they are: 1) the injury must be of a type that does not ordinarily occur unless someone was negligent; 2) the conduct that caused the injury must have been under the exclusive control of the defendant; 3) the plaintiff must not have contributed to his own injury.

8. Statute of Limitations A plaintiff who wishes to sue a defendant for an injury must do so within a specified period of time known as the *statute of limitations*. The time limit varies from state to state. Generally the statute of limitations for a tort action is three years. This means suit must be filed within three years of the alleged injury or the plaintiff is barred from making a later claim against the defendant.

9. Contributory Negligence The failure of the plaintiff to use the care of a reasonable prudent man in the protection of himself or his property. When this failure is a legally contributing cause to his injury, it is a complete defense to an action based on negligence, and the plaintiff cannot recover from the defendant.

10. Comparative Negligence A doctrine in the law of negligence by which the negligence of the parties is compared. It is basically an apportionment of damages where the degree of negligence of the plaintiff and the defendant are compared and damages awarded accordingly.

11. Outrageous Conduct Conduct which shocks the sensibilities of the ordinary citizen and which goes beyond the bounds of decency and is regarded as atrocious and utterly intolerable in a civilized community; or, it is the intentional infliction of mental or emotional distress.

Section B   Answers to True/False Items:

1. True	11. False
2. True	12. False
3. False	13. True
4. True	14. False
5. True	15. False
6. False	16. False
7. True	17. False
8. False	18. True
9. True	19. True
10. True	20. False

Section C   Answers to Multiple Choice Items:

1. a
2. e
3. b
4. b
5. d
6. c
7. d
8. b
9. b
10. c

11. c
12. b
13. a
14. c
15. b
16. e
17. e
18. b
19. c
20. a

GLOSSARY

LEGAL TERMS

A

Abortion   Expulsion of the fetus at a period of utero-gestation so early it has not acquired the power of sustaining an independent life.

Absolute Right   Given to the person in whom it inheres the uncontrolled dominion over the object at all times and for all purposes.

Ad Litem   For purposes of litigation.

Administrative Law   Branch of law dealing with organs of government power and prescribes in the manner of their activity.

Adversary   Litigant opponent—The opposing party in a writ or action.

Affiant   Person who makes and subscribes an affidavit.

Affidavit   A declaration or statement of facts, made voluntarily, and confirmed by oath.

Age of Majority   Statutory or legal age of adulthood.

Agency   Includes every relation in which one person acts for or represents another by latter's authority.

Agent   Person authorized by another to act for him.

Allegation   Charge, assertion.

Alter Ego   Second self.

Appeal   A complaint to a superior court to reverse or correct an injustice done or an alleged error committed by an inferior court.

Appellant   One taking an appeal.

Appellate Court   That court in which judgments of trial courts are reviewed or appealed.

Appellee   Party against whom appeal is taken.

Arbitrator   Neutral person chosen by both sides to decide disputed issues.

Arbitrary   Done without adequate determining principle, not done or acting according to reason.

Assault   Threat to do bodily harm.

Authority   Legal power, control over, jurisdiction.

B

Battery   Committing bodily harm.

Binding Arbitration   Submission of disputed matters for final determination.

Bona Fide   Good faith.

Borrowed Servant   An employee temporarily under the control of another. The traditional example is that of a nurse employed by a hospital who is "borrowed" by a surgeon in the operating room. The temporary employer of the borrowed servant will be held responsible for the act(s) of the borrowed servant under the doctrine of respondeat superior.

Breach of Contract   Unjustified failure to perform the terms of a contract as agreed upon or when performance is due.

C

Capricious   Willful, deliberate; done in nonrational manner, at one's pleasure.

Captain of the Ship Doctrine   Person in charge may be held responsible for all those under his supervision and makes the final decision.

Case Law   Decisions by the courts.

Cause of Action   Averment of allegations or facts sufficient to cause defendant to respond to allegations.

Caveat   Warning, beware.

Charter   The basic document which creates a corporation.

Civil Law   Concerned with the legal rights and duties of private persons.

Civil Malpractice   Professional misconduct involving a criminal act.

Client   Person who retains or employs an attorney to represent him in legal proceedings.

Common Law   Derived from court decisions, judge made law.

Comparative Negligence   Doctrine of negligence of the plaintiff and defendant is compared and an apportionment of damages is made based on the acts the parties are found to have committed.

Compensatory Damages   Amounts of money for proven loss.

Compos Mentis   Sound of mind; having use and control of one's mental facilities.

Confidential Communication Communications passing between persons on a fiduciary relationship who have a duty not to reveal the information.

Consent A voluntary act by which one person agrees to allow someone else to do something. For hospital purposes, consent should be in writing, with an explanation of the procedures to be performed, so that proof of consent is easy.

Constitutional Law Branch of law dealing with organization and function of government.

Contract A promissory agreement between two or more persons that create, modify, or destroy a legal relation. Also, it is a legally enforceable promise between two or more persons to do or not to do something.

Contract Law Law which deals with promissory agreement between two or more persons creating a legal relation.

Contributory Negligence The act or omission amounting to want of ordinary care on the part of complaining party, which, concurring with defendant's negligence, is proximate cause of injury.

Corporate Negligence Doctrine Means the hospital as an entity is negligent. It is the failure of those entrusted with the task of providing the accommodations and facilities to carry out the purpose of the corporation and the failure to follow, in a given situation, the established standards of conduct to which the corporation should conform.

Corroboration To strengthen, to add weight of credibility to a thing by additional and confirming facts or evidence.

Crime An action or offense against society as a whole.

Criminal Law Deals with conduct offensive to society as a whole, or the state.

Criminal Malpractice Professional misconduct involving a criminal act.

Cross Examination   Examination of witness upon his evidence given in chief, to test its truth or credibility.

Culpably   Blamable, censurable, connotes fault.

Cui Bono   For whose best interest, for whose good; for whose use or benefit for what good, for what useful purpose.

D

Death   Termination of life.

De Facto   In fact, actually, reality; thus, an office, position, or status existing under a claim or color of right.

Defamation   Offense of injuring another's reputation by false and malicious statements.

Defendant   In a criminal case, the person accused of committing a crime. In a civil suit, the defendant is the party against whom suit is brought.

Defense Counsel   Attorney who offers evidence as reasons in law or facts.

De Jure   By act of law.

Deposition   An oral interrogation answering all manner of questions relating to the transaction at issue, given under oath and taken in writing before some judicial officer or attorney.

Directed Verdict   Evidence presented by plaintiff is insufficient to have case go to jury and case is dismissed.

Disfranchise   To deprive of the rights and privileges of a free citizen.

Due Care   That degree of care or concern that would or should be exercised by an ordinary person in the same situation.

Due Process   Certain procedural requirements to assure fairness.

E

Emancipated The individual is no longer under the control of another.

Emergency A threat to the life or heaith of an individual that is sudden and immediate.

Equity Court Administers justice according to sense of fairness.

Ethics The science relating to moral action or moral value.

Ethical Malpractice Professional misconduct considered improper or immoral by the profession as a whole.

Euthansia Easy and painless death.

Evidentiary Matter Any species of proof, or probative matter presented by the act of the parties for the purpose of inducing belief in the minds of the court or jury as to their contention.

F

False Imprisonment Restraining another's freedom of movement without proper authority.

Fiduciary Position of trust.

Foreseeability, Doctrine of Individual is liable for all natural and proximate consequences of any negligent acts to another individual to whom a duty is owed.

Fraudulent Concealment Hiding or suppression of a material fact or circumstances which the party is legally or morally bound to disclose.

G

Genocide Mass killing of defective or handicapped human beings.

Guardian Ad Litem Is a guardian appointed to prosecute or defend a suit on behalf of a party incapacitated by infancy or otherwise.

H

Habeas Corpus   To have the body. It is a petition for release where an individual is unjustly or illegally detained or confined.

Hearsay Evidence   Evidence not proceeding from the personal knowledge of the witness.

H.M.O.   Health Maintenance Organization.

I

Iatrogenesis   Produced inadvertently as a result of treatment by a physician for some other disorder.

Indemnified   Made whole again; reimbursed.

Informed Consent   One in which the patient has received sufficient information concerning the health care proposed, its incumbent risks and the acceptable alternatives.

Injunction   A court order to stop a party to the contract from performing the specific promise or act under other circumstances.

Imputed   Ascribed vicariously to person.

Inter Alia   Among other things.

Invasion of Privacy   The right to be "left alone" to live in seclusion without being subjected to unwarranted or undesired publicity.

Involuntary Manslaughter   The unintentional taking of human life while committing an unlawful act.

J

Jurisdiction   The court has the authority to hear the case.

L

Law   The sum total of man-made rules and regulations by which society is governed in a formal and legally binding manner.

Legal   Permitted or authorized by law.

Liability   An obligation one has incurred or might incur through any act or failure to act, responsibility for conduct falling below a certain standard which is the causal connection of the plaintiff's injury.

Libel   Defamatory words that are printed, written or published which affect the character or reputation of another in that it tends to hold him up to ridicule, contempt, shame, disgrace or to degrade him in the estimation of the community.

Litigation   A trial in court to determine legal issues and the rights and duties between the parties.

Lower Court (Inferior Court)   Court which has limited authority.

M

Malpractice   Professional misconduct, improper discharge of professional duties or a failure to meet the standard of care by a professional which results in harm to another.

Mandate   Command or direction which is properly authorized and person is bound to obey.

Manslaughter   The unlawful taking of a human life without malice.

Medical Audit   A study of the patient's medical record for the purpose of determining the quality of medical care the patient received.

Medical Record   A written official documentary of what has happened to a particular patient during a specific period of time.

Mitigation   Abatement or diminution of penalty imposed by law.

Moral   Normatively human, what is expected of humans, that which they ought to do.

Mutual Assent   Clear understanding between or among parties considering an offer; known at law as a meeting of the minds.

Murder   Unlawful killing of a human being by another with malice aforethought, either express or implied.

N

Natural Death Act   The withdrawal of lifesustaining procedures from adult patients with a terminal condition where the patient has executed a "living will."

Negligence   Failure to act as an ordinary prudent person; conduct contrary to that of a reasonable person under specific circumstances.

Nominal Damages   Token compensation where the plaintiff has proven his case but the actual injury or loss is not possible to prove.

Non Compos Mentis   Not of sound mind.

O

Offeree   One who accepts an offer.

Offeror   One who makes an offer.

Outrageous Conduct, Doctrine of   That conduct which is beyond all possible bounds of decency and is regarded as atrocious and utterly intolerable in a civilized community.

P

Paramour   Illicit lover.

Parens Patrial   Duty of state to protect its citizens.

Perpetrator   Person who commits a crime, or by whose agency the act occurs.

Plaintiff   The party who brings a civil suit seeking damages or other legal relief.

Policies   Guidelines within which employees of an institution must operate.

Power of Attorney   An instrument authorizing another to act as one's agent.

Precedent   A previous adjudged decision which serves as authority in a similar case.

Prima Facie   So far as can be judged from the first disclosure; on the first appearance. A prima facie case is presented when all the necessary elements of a valid cause of action are alleged to exist. The actual existence of such facts is then subject to proof and defense at trial.

Punitive Damages   Money damages relating to punishment, and imposed as a penalty.

Privileged Communication   Statements made to one in a position of trust, usually an attorney, physician, or spouse. Because of the confidential nature of the information, the law protects it from being revealed, even in court.

Probable Cause for Arrest   More than a suspicion, but less than a certainty that a crime has been committed by a particular person.

Probate   Proving wills or handling estates.

Procedures   Mode of proceeding by which a legal right is enforced. A series of steps outlined by the institution to accomplish a specific objective or task.

Profession   The act of professing, collective body of persons in a profession.

Proximate Cause   Legal concept of cause and effect; the injury would not have occurred but for the particular cause; causal connection.

P.S.R.O.   Professional Standards Review Organization.

Pre-emptive   A right to the exclusion of others.

Preponderance   Greater weight of evidence or evidence which is more credible and convincing to the mind.

Punitive Damages   Money awarded as a penalty, damages relating to punishment.

Q

Qualified Right   Gives the possessor a right for certain purposes or under certain circumstances only.

Quid Pro Quo   Something for something.

R

Raison D'Etre   Reason for being.

Reasonable Care   That degree of skill and knowledge customarily used by a competent health practitioner or student of similar education and experience in treating and caring for the sick and injured in the community in which the individual is practicing.

Reasonably Prudent Man Doctrine   Requires a person of ordinary sense to use ordinary care and skill.

Rebuttal   Introduction of evidence to show statement of witness is not credible.

Redress   Satisfaction for the injury sustained.

Remand   Send back.

Res Ipsa Loquitur   "The thing speaks for itself." A doctrine of law applicable to cases where the defendant had exclusive control of the thing which caused the harm and where the harm ordinarily could not have occurred without negligent conduct. Normally, the plaintiff must prove the defendant's liability but when this doctrine is found to apply, the defendant must prove himself not responsible for harm.

Respondeat Superior   "Let the master answer." The employer is responsible for the legal consequences of the acts of the servant or employee while he acts within the scope of his employment.

Respondent   The person who argues against a petition or appeal, generally the person who prevailed in the lower court, the appellee.

Right   Power, privilege or faculty inherent in one person and incident upon another.

Rules and Regulations   Clear and concise statements mandating or prohibiting certain activity in an institution.

Rule of Discovery   Statute of limitations does not begin to run until the patient knew or should have known of the injury.

Reasonable Doubt   Ordinary or usual knowledge of facts of a character calculated to induce a doubt in the mind of an ordinarily intelligent and prudent businessman.

S

Sacrosanct   Not to be violated.

Sequester   Setting apart, to isolate witnesses.

Signatory   One who signs.

Slander   Speaking falsely about another with resulting inquiry to his reputation.

Standard of Care   Those acts performed or omitted that an ordinary prudent person in the defendant's position would have done or not done; a measure by which the defendant's conduct is compared to ascertain negligence.

Standard of Reasonableness   Measures how the average ordinary prudent individual is expected to act in certain circumstances.

Standards   Criteria of measuring, and conformity to established practice.

Statute of Limitations   A legal limit on the time one has to file suit in civil matters, usually measured from the time of the wrong or from the time a reasonable man would have discovered the wrong.

Statutes Legislative enactments; act of legislature declaring, commanding or prohibiting something.

Statutory Law Enacted by a legislative group.

Subpoena A court order requiring one to come to court to give testimony; failure to appear results in punishment by the court.

Subpoena Duces Tecum Bring the documents.

Sui Juris Of his own right; possessing full social and civil rights; not under any legal disability, or the power of another, or guardianship; having capacity to manage one's own affairs.

Sua Sponte Of his or its own will or motion; voluntarily; without prompting or suggestion.

Suit Court proceeding where one person seeks damages or other legal remedies from another. The term is not usually used in connection with criminal cases.

Superior Court Court of the highest and most extensive jurisdiction.

Symbiotic Relationship Mutually dependent relationship.

T

Taft-Hartley Act Enacted in 1947 by Congress, considered a pro-management law. It excluded non-profit hospitals from Federal coverage.

Tort A legal or civil wrong committed by one person against the person or property of another.

Transsexual An obsession to belong to the opposite sex which is not practically reversible by psychological or other medical treatment.

Transvestite A person who wears clothing appropriate to the opposite sex and who desires to be accepted as a member of the opposite sex.

U

Uniform Commercial Code Statutory enactments which govern business transactions and that are uniformly accepted from state to state.

Unit of Employees A group of two or more who share common employment interest and conditions.

V

Verdict The formal declaration of the jury of its findings of fact, which is signed by the jury foreman and presented to the court.

Verdict of Acquittal Argument that there is not sufficient evidence against the defendant to proceed and the case should be dismissed.

Viability Capability of living, term to denote the power a newborn infant possesses to independently exist.

Vicarious—Substitute.

Viz That is to say; contraction for videlicet, to wit, namely.

Void Having no legal force.

Voluntary Manslaughter Taking of human life in the heat of passion when suddenly provoked.

W

Wagner Act First national labor relations act enacted in 1935 to protect workers' right to organize and elect their own representative.

Waived   Renounce or give up a privilege.

Witnessing   One who testifies to what he has seen, heard or otherwise observed.

Writ   A writing issuing from a court ordering a sheriff or other officer of the law or some other person to perform an action desired by the court or authorizing an action to be done.

BIBLIOGRAPHY

Accreditation Manual for Hospitals, Joint Commission on Hospital Accreditation, Chicago, Illinois, December, 1970.

ACKERMAN, S. N., "No Fault Insurance Could Relieve Malpractice Pressure": *Modern Hospitals,* September, 1970, 115 (3), P. 112-4.

ADDENNBROOKE, DR. F. CLARKE, Letter: "Confidentiality of Medical Records," *British Medical Journal,* 1 (5948): 39, 4 January, 1975.

BENSOUSSAN, P. A., *Modern Drug Addiction: Present Condition in 1972 in the U.S.A.,* Ann. Med. Pschol. July–August, 1972.

BERNSTEIN, ARTHUR, "Staff Privileges and the Hospital's Liability to Patients," *Hospitals, JAHA,* Vol. 47, pp. 156-170, March, 1973.

BERNSTEIN, A. H., "Of Hospitals, Negligence, and Contracts," *Hospitals, JAHA,* August, 1973, 47 (15): P. 120-122.

BERNSWEIG, ELI P., *Legal Aspects of PHY Medical Care,* PHSP No. 1468, U.S. Government Printing Office, 1966.

BERNSWEIG, ELI P., *The Problems of Medical Malpractice as Viewed by the Federal Government in Report First National Conference on Medical Malpractice,* 22, Feb. 7–8, 1970.

BLAES, STEPHEN, "Why and How Should Bylaws be Revised," *Hospitals, J.A.H.A.,* Vol. 47, pp. 100-106, December, 1973.

BLUM, RICHARD H., *The Management of the Doctor-Patient Relationship,* McGraw-Hill Book Co. New York, 1960.

BUSH, VANESSA. "New Data Battle: State's Need to Know vs. Patient's Privacy," *Modern Health Care,* May, 1975.

Child Abuse Prevention and Treatment Act, Act of January 31, 1974, Pub. Law No. 93-247; 88 Stat 4 (1973).

Children's Bureau, U.S. Dept. of Health, Education and Welfare, *The*

Abused Child—Principles and Suggested Language for Legislation on Reporting of the Physically Abused Child (1963).

CLELAND, VIRGINIA S., "Supervisor in Collective Bargaining," *Journal of Nursing Administration.* 4:33-35, Sept.–Oct. 1974.

COHEN, IRA A., "Medical and Dental Malpractice," PLI, 1969, New York City.

CROSSLAND, JANICE. "Human Experimentation," *Nursing Digest,* May–June, 1975, pp. 33-35.

CURRAN, WILLIAM J. *Law, Medicine and Forensic Science,* 2nd Ed. (Little, Brown and Co., Boston, 1970).

CURRAN, W. J., E. M. LASKA, H. KAPLAN, R. BANK, "Protection of Privacy and Confidentiality," *Science,* 182 (114): 797-892, November 1973.

DRISCO I, VERONICA M., "Myth of Two Hats: Nursing Service Director in the Collective Bargaining Situation," *Supervisor Nurse,* 5:24-27, June 1974.

Early Childhood Project Education Commission, *Child Abuse and Neglect: Model Legislation for the States* (1973).

FRIEDMAN, S. B., "The Need for Intensive Follow-Up of Abused Children." *Helping the Battered Child and His Family,* C. Henry Kempe and Ray E. Helfer, Lippincott Co., Philadelphia, PA, 1972.

FROST, HAROLD A. and AUSUBEL, MARVIN, *Preparation of a Negligence Case,* PLI, 1970, New York City.

GAIR, HARRY A. and CONASON, ROBERT, *The Trail of a Negligence Action,* PLI, 1970, New York City.

GOLDBERG, JOEL H., "The Extraordinary Confusion Over the Right to Die," *Medical Economics,* January 10, 1977, P. 122.

GOODMAN, RICHARD M., *Modern Hospital Liability: Law and Tactics,* PLI, 1971, New York City.

GREGORY, CHARLES, *Cases and Materials on Torts,* 2nd Ed. (Little, Brown and Co., 1970).

HAYT & HAYT, *Law of Hospital and Nurses,* Hospital Textbook Co., New York, New York, 1958.

HERSHEY, N., "The Defensive Practice of Medicine: Myth or Reality," *Milbank Memorial Fund Quarterly,* January, 1972, 50 (1): pp. 69-98.

HERSHEY, NATHAN. "An Alternative to Mandatory Licensure of Health Professions," *Hospital Progress,* Vol. 50, Marcy 1969, P. 71.

"History of Medical Record Science," *Medical Record News,* October, 1969, Vol. 40, No. 5.

HOBBS, T., "Fire, Pestilence, Blood and Medical Malpractice Suits,"

Journal of the Medical Association of the State of Alabama, March, 1974, 43 (9): pp. 541-42 Passim.

HOFFMAN, C. A., "International Aspects of Malpractice," *Internal Surgery, February,* 1974, 59 (2): pp. 78-80.

HOLDER, A. R., "Medical Premises Liability," *JAMA,* November, 1973, 226 (6): pp. 717-8.

HOLDER, A. R., "Creation of the Physician—Patient Relationship," *JAMA,* December 10, 1973, 226 (11): pp. 1391-92.

HOLDER, A. R., "Recent Decisions of Emergency Room Liability," *JAMA,* March 4, 1974, 227 (9): pp. 1087-89.

HOLDER, A. R., "The Physician As Rescuer," *JAMA,* February 5, 1973, 223 (6): pp. 721-22.

HORTY, JOHN F., "Who Says It's An Emergency?" *Modern Health Care,* May, 1975.

HURT, T., "Principles of Tort Liability and Elements of Emergency Health Care for Educators: A Self-Instructional Text Developed Through the Use of a Systems Model and Intrinsic Programming," Journal of School Health, June, 1973, 43 (6): pp. 345-49.

Kansas Statutes Annotated, Sec. 77-202 Supp. 1971.

KARST, KENNETH L., "The Files: Legal Controls Over the Accuracy and Accessibility of Stored Personal Data," Professor of Law, University of California, Los Angeles.

KELLY, LUCIE, "Nursing Practice Acts," *American Journal of Nursing,* July, 1974, p. 1310-1319.

KELLY, LUCIE YOUNG, "Institutional Licensure," *Nursing Outlook,* 21:666, 570, Sept. 1973.

KEPLER, M. O., "The Abuse of Drug Abuse," *Clinical Pediatrics,* July, 1972.

KETCHAM, ORMAN W., PAULSEN, MONRAD G., *Cases and Materials Relating to Juvenile Courts,* The Foundation Press, 1967.

KING, J. Y., "A Critique of the Report of HEW's Medical Malpractice Commission," (University of Maryland Legal Law School), *Journal of Legal Medicine,* March–April, 1974, 2 (2): 49-54.

KRAMER, CHARLES, *Medical Malpractice,* PLI, 1971, New York City.

Lawyer's Medical Journal, The Lawyers Co-Operative Publishing Co., New York.

Legal Medicine, Vol. 5, No. 4 (April, 1977), pp. 17-24.

LELLOGG, NED, "Suddenly, Nurses Can Bargain for Professional Goals," *RN,* Library Edition, 37:43+, Sept. 1974.

LIPMAN, M., "Can You Afford to be a Good Samaritan? Yes!," *R.N.,* September, 1974, 37 (9): 90-91.

LOCKHART, KAMISAR & CHAPER, *Constitutional Rights and Liberties,* West Publishing Co., St. Paul, Minn., 1968.

LONG, EDNA S., "How to Survive Hospitalization," *American Journal of Nursing,* March, 1974.

LOUISELL, D. and WILLIAMS, H., *Trial of Medical Malpractice Cases,* Matthew Bender & Co., 1966.

McCABE, J. J.: McCABE, J. J., "What to Do if You are Sued for Malpractice," *Journal of Legal Medicine,* May–June, 1974, 2 (3): 21-25.

McCORMICK, RICHARD, *Ambiguity in Moral Choice.* The 1973 Pere Marquette Theology Lecture, Milwaukee: Marquette University Theology Publication, 1973.

McNULTY, ELIZABETH, "How Survey Mechanism Works," *Hospitals, JAHA,* Vol. 45, July 1, 1971, pp. 36-40.

MACKERT, MARY ELLEN, "JCAH Standards Generate Goals," *Hospital, JAHA,* Vol. 47, pp. 85-89, January, 1973.

MAGUIRE, DANIEL, *Death by Choice,* (Doubleday and Company, Inc. Garden City, New York, 1974), P. 77.

"Medical Adversity Insurance: A No-Fault Approach to Medical Malpractice and Quality Assurance," *Milbank Memorial Fund Quarterly,* Spring, 1973, 51 (2): 125-168.

Medico-Legal Brief: "Physician Liability for Health Care Assistants," *Journal of the Mississippi State Medical Association,* February, 1974, 15 (2): 64.

MILLS, DON H., "Malpractice and the Administration of Drugs," *Medical Times,* 93:657 (June, 1965).

National Symposium on Child Abuse Presented in Rochester, New York, October 19, 1971.

"On Cerebral, Brain, Systemic Death," In Current Concepts of Cerebrovascular Disease: *Stroke,* A publication of the American Heart Association, Inc. 8, No. 3 (May–June 1973):9.

PRESSER, C. S.: "Legal Problems Attendant to Sex Reassignment Surgery."

PROSSER, WILLIAM, *Handbook of the Law of Torts,* St. Paul: West Publishing Co., 3rd Ed. 1964.

Public Law No. 93-247, Section 4(b) (2) (B).

RAMSEY, PAUL, *The Patient As Person* (New Haven and London: Yale University Press, 1970), P. 162.

Report of the Secretary's Advisory Committee on Automated Personal Data Systems, *Record Computers and the Rights of Citizens,* Department of Health, Education and Welfare Publication, July, 1973.

Report of the Secretary's Commission on Medical Malpractice, Washington, D.C. Dept. of Health, Education and Welfare, No. (05) 73-88, 1973.

Restatement of Torts (2nd edition), Section 46, 1965.

RIBICOFF, "Medical Malpractice: The Patient vs. The Physician" 6 Trail 10 (1970).

ROBERTS, BRUCE, "Accreditation and Legality, *AORN Journal*, Vol. 14, pp. 49-52, September, 1971.

ROSASCO, LOUISE C., "Collective Bargaining: What's a Director of Nursing to Do?" *Hospital, J.A.H.A.*, 48-79+, September 16, 1974.

ROSS, ELISABETH KUBLER, *Questions and Answers on Death and Dying*, MacMillan Publishing Co. Inc., New York, 1974, pp. 76-78.

ROTHBERG, JUNE S., "Why Nursing Diagnosis?" *AJN*, 67:1040 (May, 1967).

"Statutory Brain Death?" Department of Pathology, University of Southern California, Los Angeles. *Journal of the American Medical Association*, August 26, 1974. Vol. 229, P. 87.

STEWART, BRADFORD, and KELLY, "Medical Practice, Why the Increase in Malpractice Litigation," 27 Insurance Counsel (1960).

The Best of Law and Medicine. Articles selected from the *Journal of the American Medical Association*, 1968–1970.

The Citation, American Medical Association, Chicago, IL.

Time Magazine, March 14, 1977, "Viewing Life Before Birth," p. 60.

Transsexuals in Limbo: The Search for a Legal Definition of Sex, 31 *MD Law Rev.* (1971), pp. 236-254.

VANATTA, F. A., "Electrical Hazards in Hospitals," Washington: National Academy of Sciences, 1970.

VISSCHER, MAURICE B., ed., *Humanistic Perspectives in Medical Ethics*, Buffalo: Prometheus Books, 1972.

WASSMER, THOMAS A., "Between Life and Death: Ethical and Moral Issues Involved in Recent Medical Advances," Villanova Law Review 13 (1968):776.

WEISMAN, AVERY D., On Dying and Denying, New York: Behavioral Publications, Inc., 1972.

"What You Haven't Read About the Nork Case," *Medical Economics*, July 22, 1974.

WINTER, ARTHUR, ed., *The Moment of Death*, Illinois: Charles C. Thomas Co., Inc., 1969.

WUNDERLICH, R. A., "Pattern of Multiple Drug Abuse Among Adolescents Referred by a Juvenile Court," *Pediatrics*. June, 1971.

ZEBROWSKI, DELORES, "Collective Bargaining and the Director of Nursing," *Supervisor Nurse*, 5:16, June, 1974.

Cases

1. *Bartley v. Kremens*, 402 F. Supp. 1039 (E.D. Pa. 1975), Prob. Juris noted, 96 S. Ct. 1457 (1976).
2. *Bernardi v. Community Hospital Association*, 443 P. 2d 708 (1968).
3. *Carroll v. Kittle*, 457 P. 2d 21 (Kansas, 1964).
4. *Cobbs v. Grant*, 104, 229 Cal. RPTR. 505, 502 P. 2d 1 (1972).
5. *Cohen v. New York*, 382 NYS, 2d 128 (New York, 1975).
6. *Cunningham v. MacNeal Memorial Hospital*, 251 N.E. 2d 733 (1969).
7. *Coe v. Gerstein*, 376 F. Supp., 695 (S.D. Fla., 1974).
8. *Darling v. Charleston Community Hospital*, 211 N.E. 2d 253 (1965).
9. *Doe v. Bolton*, 410 U.S. 179, (1973).
10. *Doe v. Poelker*, 515 F. 2d 541 (1973).
11. *DiRosse v. Wein*, 261 N.Y.S. 2d 623.
12. *Finn v. City of New York*, 335 NY, 2d 516 (1972).
13. *Fiorentino v. Wenger*, 19 N.Y. 2d 407 (1967).
14. *Gray v. Grunnagle*, 233 A2d 663 (1966).
15. *Griswold v. Connecticut*, 381 U.S. 479, 85 S. Ct. 1678 (1975).
16. *Helman v. Sacred Heart Hospital*, 62 Wash. 2d 136 (1963).
17. *Johnson v. Woman's Hospital*, 527 S.U. 3rd 133 (Tenn. App., 1975).
18. *Keeler v. Superior Court*, 2 Col. 3d 619 (1970).
19. *Landeros v. Glood*, 131 Cal. RPTR 69, 551 P. 2d 389 (1976).
20. *McDowell Hospital v. Minks*, 529 So. 2d 360 (Kentucky, 1975).
21. *Martin v. Bralliar*, 540 P. 2d 1118 (Colorado App., 1975).
22. *Meyer v. Nottiger*, 241 NoW. 2d 911 (Iowa, 1976).
23. *Mitchell v. Robinson*, 344 S.W. 2d 11.
24. *Mundt v. Alta Bates Hospital*, 35 Col. RPTR. 848 (1963).
25. *Murray v. Vondevander*, 522 P. 2d 302 (IL. App., 1974).
26. *Nance v. James Archer*, Smith Hospital, Inc., 329 So. 2d 377 (Fla. App., 1976).
27. *Newhall v. Central Vermont Hospital*, 349 A. 2d 890 (VT. 1975).
28. *Norton v. Argonaut Insurance Co.*, 144 So. 2d 249 (1962).
29. *Pegram v. Sisco*, 406 F. Supp. 776 (D. Ark. 1976).
30. *People v. Chavez*, 77 Col. App. 2d 621 (1970).
31. *Robinson v. California*, 370 U.S. 660 (1962).

32.   *Roe v. Wade,* 410 U.S. 113 (1973).

33.   *Schloendorf v. Soc. of New York Hosp.,* 211 N.Y. 125, 105 N.E. 92 (1974).

34.   *Schields v. King,* 3 17 N.E. 2d 922 (Ohio App., 1973).

35.   *Wilmington General Hospital v. Manlove,* 174 A2d 135 (1961).

INDEX

Abortion, 3, 19, 51, 68
  and indigent patients, 3
  Supreme Court decisions, 69
Abuse (*see* Child abuse)
Actual damages (*see* Compensatory damages)
Administrative law, 193
Adversary proceeding, 4, 5
AFL-CIO, 176
Ally doctrine, 56
American Hospital Association, 66
Appeal procedure, 199
Appellate court, 18
Appropriate bargaining unit, 54
Arrest, definition, 186
Assault and battery, 8, 10, 13
Authority, 200-202
  legal definition, 200
Automated record keeping (*see* Computers)

Bader v. United Orthodox Synagogue, 107
Bailment, 165
Bargaining units, of hospital, 54
  (*see also* Appropriate bargaining unit)
Bartley v. Kremens, 103
Battered child syndrome, 13, 76, 79
Battery, definition, 10
Borrowed servant doctrine, 26, 211
Breach of contract, 46
  (*see also* Contracts)

Captain of the ship doctrine, 27
Cardiopulmonary resuscitation, 174
Cause of action, 7
  four elements, 14
Charles v. U.S., 185

Child abuse, 72, 75, 77, 104
and neglect, 74
sexual, 78
Child Abuse Prevention and
Treatment Act, 73, 78
Children
child labor laws, 73
mental health care, 103
minors (*see* Minors)
Children's Bureau Report (1963),
73
Circuit courts, 195
Civil law system, 6, 7, 191
Civil malpractice, 13
Civil suits, procedure, 15
Code of Hammurabi, 61
Coe v. Gerstein, 71
Cohen v. New York, 36
Collective bargaining, 53
Common law system, 6, 191
Comparative negligence, 41, 212
Compensatory damages, 43
Computers, and confidentiality,
125
Confidentiality, 104, 111, 112, 125
of medical records, 106-109,
118-120
and news media, 108
release of information, 126
Consent, 90, 91, 94-97, 135
and emergency, 94
informed consent, 90, 94, 96-97
of spouse, 92
Consideration, 46
Constitutional law, 193
Contracts, 44, 153
breach of contract, 46
classifications, 48
contract law, 192
defined, 44
elements of, 45
nurses, 50-51
oral, 48

Contributory negligence, 41, 212
(*see also* Negligence)
Coronary Care Unit, 176
Corporations
corporate negligence, 31-32, 114
formed by doctors, 27
Countersigning, 117, 133
Court system, 195-197
functions, 15
Crime
definition, 6
criminal law, 6, 192
Cross-examination, 5

Damages, 12, 14, 18, 40
compensatory damages, 43
nominal damages, 43
*Darling v. Charleston Community
Hospital,* 21, 31
Death, 81-85, 148-149
definition of, 84
heroic measures, 148-149
wills, 166-167
Defamation of character, 9
Depotism, 16-17
Discovery rule, 15, 42
Doctrine of outrageous conduct,
39
Doe v. Bolton, 69
Doe v. Poelker, 3
Drugs (*see* Medication)
Due care, 13
Due process, 102

Early Childhood Project Education Commission, 73
Emancipation, of minors, 93
Emergency, 175
emergency admission, 101
emergency room, 183
Emotional distress, 39
Equipment, 156
defective equipment, 155

Equipment (*cont.*)
  routine check, 38
  warranty, 37-38
Equity court, definition, 47
Ethical malpractice, 13
Euthanasia, 12, 81, 86-87
Evidence, 6, 17
  evidentiary matter, 91
Exigency, 9

False imprisonment, 9
Federal judicial system, 195
Fiduciary duty, 94
First Amendment, 145-146
Foreseeability, 212
Fourth Amendment, 184
Fraud, 9-10

Gonzales v. Nork, 33, 114
Griswold v. Connecticut, 69
Grievance procedures, 57-58
Guardian, 73

Habeus corpus, definition, 103
*Hammonds v. Aetna Casualty and
  Surety Company,* 109
Hemodyalysis, 35
Heroic measures, 148-149
Homosexual, 98
Horne v. Patton, 109
Hospitals
  admission, 101
  bargaining units, 54
  leaving against advice, 139-141
  teaching hospitals, 150-151
Hypodermic injection, 8
Hysterectomy, 100

Iatrogenesis, 114
Incompetent staff, 143
Indemnification, 25
Indigent patients, 3

Information
  and confidentiality, 105-107,
    109
  interchange between profes-
    sionals, 110
Injunction, 47
Insulin, 25
Insurance, 171, 172-173, 175
Intensive Care Unit, 160, 172, 175,
    203
Intent, 8
Intentional torts, 7
International Commission of Jus-
    tice (1970), 104
Involutionary commitment, 101
Irradiation, and iatrogenics, 114

Johnson v. Woman's Hospital, 39
Joint Commission on Accredita-
    tion of Hospitals, 113

Kamikaze pilots, 82
Kruszewski v. Holz-May, 99

Labor relations, 53, 175, 194
Landeros v. Flood, 77
Landmark decisions, 23
Law
  classifications, 194-195
  definition, 3
  origin of, 5
Legal proceedings, guidelines,
    187-189
Legal terms, 221-235
Legislation, lag, 21
Liability, 12, 18, 26, 49
  borrowed servant doctrine, 26,
    27
  and confidentiality, 108-109
  corporate negligence, 31
  doctrine of foreseeability, 36
  of hospital, 32
  no-fault insurance, 28

Liability (*cont.*)
  and negligence, 180-181
  and medication, 182-183
  of nurse, 97
  personal liability, 22, 211
  personal property, 164-166
  in psychiatric care, 37
  reasonably prudent man, 28
  doctrine of respondent superior,
    24, 158
  res ipsa loquitur doctrine, 34-35
  and supervision, 157
  warranty, 37
Libel, 9

Majority exclusive representative
    principle, 55
Malpractice law, 11, 12, 20-21, 171
  classifications, 12
  insurance, 173
  no-fault insurance, 28
  prima facie case, 14
  Secretary's Commission on
    Medical Malpractice, 112
Manslaughter, definition, 7
Mapp v. Ohio, 185
McDowell Hospital v. Minks, 30
Medical acts, 46
Medical malpractice law, 194
Medical mystique, 19
Medication
  administration, 14, 20, 127, 162,
    182
  illegible medication orders, 138-
    39
  and malpractice, 14
  procurement, 46
  refusal to administer, 127
  splitting medication, 152-153
Mental capacity, 101
Mental competence, 46
Mental health care, 102-103, 127
  commitment laws, 128

Mental health care (*cont.*)
  liability, 37
  voluntary commitment, 127
Meyer v. Nottger, 39
Minors, 42
  medical records, 120
  mental health care, 103
Misfeasance, 129
Money damages (*see* Damages)
Murder, 82
  definition, 7
Murray v. Vandevander, 93
Mutual assent, 45

*Nance v. James Archer Smith
    Hospital,* 38
National Center for Prevention of
    Child Abuse and Neglect, 75
National Labor Relations Act, 53
National Labor Relations Board,
    54-55, 176
Negligence, 11, 158, 180-181
  comparative, 41
  contributory, 41
  doctrine of corporate negli-
    gence, 31, 211
  and malpractice, 11
  Nork case, 33, 114
*Newhall v. Central Vermont Hos-
    pital,* 29
News media, and confidentiality,
    108, 160
No-fault insurance, 28
Nominal damages, 43
Nuremburg code, 70
Nurses
  administration of medication,
    163, 182-183
  charge nurses, 121
  Director of Nurses, 203
  guidelines for legal problems,
    187-189
  liability, 23, 24, 97

Nurses (*cont.*)
  license, 7
  practitioners, 20
  records, 114-115
  students, 131-132

Oral contracts, 48
Outrageous conduct, 40, 212

Paren patriae doctrine, 93
Patient's rights (*see* Rights of patients)
Pennsylvania Mental Health and Retardation Act, 103
Pension plans, 53
Perjury, 17
Personal liability, 22
Pharmacy Act, 163
Police power, 178, 179
Power of attorney, 92
Precedent, 191
Privacy, 104, 112, 145, 161
Privileged communication statutes, 111
Proximate cause, 13
Physician's assistants, 20
Prima facie case, 14, 15

Quid pro quo, 46, 49
Quinlan case, 84, 87-88

Reasonable care, 11
Reasonableness, 10, 20, 30
  reasonably prudent man doctrine, 28, 30, 211
Records, 112, 120
  (*see also* Information)
  access, 111, 119
  alteration, 118
  classification, 106
  and computers, 125-126
  countersigning, 134-135
  and minors, 120

Records (*cont.*)
  and privacy, 107-109
  purposes, 113
Redress, 9, 40
Refusal of treatment, 97
Res ipsa loquitur, 212
Respondent superior doctrine, 24, 158, 211
Restraints, 128-129
Resuscitation, 146-147
Rights, 65
  definition, 61
  health care rights, 61-63
  of patients, 3, 62-63
    of indigent patients, 3
    Minnesota statute, 65
    patient's bill of rights, 66-67
  of private persons, 7
Risk management, 171
Roe v. Wade, 69
Rule of discovery (*see* Discovery rule)

Safe practice, 20
Sanctity of life principle, 83
Schloendorf v. Society of New York Hospital, 137
Search and seizure, 183-185
Secondary boycott, 56
Secretary's Commission on Medical Malpractice, 112
Sex reassignment surgery, 98
Sexual abuse, 78
Shields v. King, 35
Shock Trauma Emergency Unit, 176
Slander, 9
Social Security Act, 3
Society, and law, 3
Society for the Right to Die, 81
Standards
  of care
    definition, 12

Standards *(cont.)*
  of care *(cont.)*
    establishment, 13
    customs and usage, 22
State Board of Examiners, 188
State Nurses' Association, 176
Statute of Limitations, 16, 42, 212
Statute of Frauds, 44, 48
Statutory law, definition, 5
Sterile technique, 4
Stimulus, and perception, 5
Students, 131
Suicide, 37
Supervision, 157, 177
  defined by NLRB, 177
  role of supervisor, 55
Supreme Court, 3, 4, 69, 184
Surgery
  and battery, 8
  transexual, 98, 99

Taft-Hartley Act, 53
Teamsters, 176
Testimony, 5
Thantology, 81
Tort law
  elements of, 13
  and emotional distress, 39

Tort law *(cont.)*
  false imprisonment, 9
  and health professionals, 10
  intentional torts, 7
  and malpractice, 11
  and negligence, 7, 8
Transvestite, 98
Transexual, 98
Trial procedure, 199

Uniform Business Records as Evidence Act, 120
Uniform Commercial Code, 194
Unions, 53, 176
United States of America v. Martha L. Woods, 79
U. S. Constitution, 3

Warrants, 185
Warranty, 37
Watergate hearings, 5
Wills, 166-167
  definition, 169
  signature, 170
Witness, 5, 17
  function, 16
Workmen's compensation, 178

Date Due

MAY 20 '85			
APR 24 '92			
MAR 15 '94			
MAR 25 '94			
MAR 2 5 2000			
DEC 04 2001			